CLINICAL ETHICS

ALBERT R. JONSEN, PH.D.
Professor of Ethics in Medicine,
Department of Medicine, School of Medicine,
University of California, San Francisco

MARK SIEGLER, M.D.
Associate Professor of Medicine, Department of
Medicine, Section of General Internal Medicine,
Pritzker School of Medicine, University of Chicago

WILLIAM J. WINSLADE, PH.D., J.D.
Co-Director, Program in Medicine, Law and
Human Values, Adjunct Professor of Law, School of Law, and
Adjunct Professor of Psychiatry,
School of Medicine, University of California,
Los Angeles; Research Clinical Associate,
Southern California Psychoanalytic Institute

CLINICAL ETHICS

A Practical Approach to Ethical Decisions in Clinical Medicine

Macmillan Publishing Co., Inc.
NEW YORK

Collier Macmillan Canada, Inc.
TORONTO

Collier Macmillan Publishers
LONDON

Printed in the United States of America

Macmillan Publishing Co., Inc.
866 Third Avenue, New York, New York 10022

Collier Macmillan Canada, Inc.
Collier Macmillan Publishers · London

Library of Congress Cataloging in Publication Data

Jonsen, Albert R.
Clinical ethics.

Bibliography: p.
Includes index.
1. Medical ethics. 2. Medical ethics—Case Studies.
I. Siegler, Mark. II. Winslade, William J. III. Title.
[DNLM: 1. Ethics, Medical. W 50 J81c]
R724.J66 174'.2 81-20839
ISBN 0-02-361360-2 AACR2

Printing: 5 6 7 8 Year: 5 6 7 8 0 1

The authors dedicate *Clinical Ethics* to three physicians:

Julius Krevans, M.D.,
Dean of the School of Medicine, University of California, San Francisco

Alvin R. Tarlov, M.D.,
Professor of Medicine, Department of Medicine, Pritzker School of Medicine, University of Chicago

Bernard Towers, M.B., CH.B.,
Professor of Pediatrics and Anatomy, Co-Director of the Program in Medicine, Law and Human Values, School of Medicine, University of California, Los Angeles

who have fostered their work and encouraged the conjunction of clinical involvement and philosophical reflection, the essential ingredients of clinical ethics.

FOREWORD

Despite the increasing importance of ethics in medicine, few clinicians spend the time and effort it takes to read a book on ethics. All too often these books have been couched in weighty philosophy and abstruse theory.

This little book handles ethical problems in medicine quite differently. Jointly authored by an ethicist, a clinician, and a lawyer, it attacks ethical problems in real-life terms. For example, how should a physician handle the patient who has a respiratory arrest, becomes anoxic, and never wakes up from a coma? What should be the role of the family in influencing this decision? How does the presence or absence of underlying disease affect this decision-making process?

Or, how should the physician handle the heroin addict who has had endocarditis on a prosthetic valve if he does not cease using intravenous narcotics?

Or, should an overweight diabetic who refuses to take her insulin, adhere to her diet, and take care of her foot ulcers be offered chronic dialysis when she develops renal failure?

These and many other illustrated cases provide various options that must be considered in the management of some of these difficult ethical and clinical problems. The authors provide the best advice of which they are capable.

Not all readers will agree with every piece of advice offered. In general, however, the advice the authors give is consonant with good common sense, generally accepted ethical teachings, and legal statutes.

Not only does this book provide answers to specific clinical problems, but it serves as a remarkably complete primer of medical ethics. Mainly by means of brief case illustrations, it addresses itself to such difficult issues as the decision to withdraw life support, the definition of brain death, when to order "no code," respect for patient autonomy, the contractual arrangements between physicians and patients, the question of patient competence and mental incapacity, informed consent, refusal of treatment by competent persons, confidentiality, and failure to comply with medical regimens. There is an excellent chapter on the role of the "quality of life" as it is perceived by patients and medical personnel. There are lucid discussions of euthanasia and suicide.

Although this book focuses primarily on the relationship between an individual patient and his/her physician, the last chapter deals with external factors that have ethical implications. These include the role of the family, the cost of medical care, the allocation of scarce resources, and ethical behavior in teaching and research. For me the book ends on a very upbeat note because the authors condemn the withholding of services by physicians (e.g., strikes) as unethical, a principle in which I devoutly believe.

This is a very useful little book, primarily because it is so helpful to the "working doctor." As one who is easily intimidated by legalisms and philosophical tenets, I found the practical approach taken by these authors refreshing, informative, and skillful. I certainly considered the three hours I invested in reading this brief volume well spent, and I suspect most of my colleagues who practice internal medicine will have the same reaction.

Robert G. Petersdorf, M.D., M.A.C.P.
Dean and Vice Chancellor for Health Sciences and Professor of Medicine,
University of California, San Diego,
School of Medicine, La Jolla

PREFACE

We have written this book for physicians, particularly those who practice general and internal medicine (although practitioners of other specialties, nurses, and medical students should find it helpful). We presuppose that all of our readers have some knowledge of medicine and of the clinical care of patients.

All three of us lay claim to some clinical experience as either practitioners or consultants. Each of us is trained in different disciplines: Jonsen in philosophy and moral theology; Siegler in medicine; Winslade in law, philosophy, and psychoanalysis. We came away from wards and clinics, from books and lectures, with the intention of bringing our experience and training to bear on the ethical problems facing the practitioner of medicine.

Practitioners must make decisions. Thus, we do not merely discuss or analyze the ethical problems; we offer counsel about decisions. Lest this be thought presumptuous, we do not consider our counsel the single and final answer. We offer it in the tradition of medical consultation: The consultant may bring to the practitioner's view of the case not only broader information but another perspective.

Our experience with ethical problems in clinical settings, our familiarity with the literature, and our training in various fields allow us to offer broader information about certain issues than the practitioner is likely to command. However, it was in the application of our differing perspectives to each case that we grew confident enough to offer counsel. Siegler inclined somewhat to the paternalism often associated with medicine; Winslade favored the autonomy of the patient; Jonsen stressed the application of principles to each case. Out of discussion colored by these perspectives, we reached decisions. We soon realized that these viewpoints frequently converged when practical decisions had to be made.

Although it is not possible to form a trio like ours for every ethical decision, practitioners can replay in their own minds the themes we identify as they consider which decision would be best and right. This experience leads us to offer counsel to those physicians who have neither the opportunity nor the leisure to do what we have done.

We are grateful to those who read our manuscript with a critical eye: James Childress, Ph.D.; Eugene Hildreth, M.D.; Andrew Jameton, Ph.D.; Bernard Lo, M.D.; Henry Perkins, M.D.; Judy Ross, M.A.; John Robertson, J.D.; and Daniel Wikler, Ph.D. They bear no responsibility for our faults, but much credit for our merits. We acknowledge the interest shown by the American Board of Internal Medicine in the teaching of clinical ethics. That interest stimulated the writing of this book. We also appreciate the support of the Commonwealth Fund, the Josiah Macy Foundation, and the National Endowment for the Humanities.

Albert R. Jonsen
Mark Siegler
William J. Winslade

CONTENTS

LOCATOR

* Numbers refer to sections. **Boldface numbers** indicate major treatments of the topic.

CLINICAL ETHICS

INTRODUCTION

In routine clinical practice, physicians sometimes confront problems that are referred to as ethical problems. They appear in a variety of ways. Some are of the dramatic sort reported in the newspapers: Kidneys are removed from a man who, it is alleged, was not dead; a family seeks legal authority to remove a dying parent from a respirator against their physician's advice; an elderly woman refuses permission for an amputation. Others are more commonplace: How much information should be given to a fearful patient in whom cancer is detected; how should the persistently noncompliant patient be cared for; what information should be kept confidential from the family? Every physician can relate incidents of this sort, which may be described as "ethical," even though it may not be very clear as to what makes the problem an ethical one.

All practitioners face these problems from time to time; many feel distinctly uncomfortable when they do. This discomfort stems, in part, from the nature of the problems: They often involve life-and-death decisions that engage profound human emotions and require intense and delicate dealings with other persons. In addition, discomfort may arise because physicians may feel they have not been trained to approach such problems systematically. Methods of analyzing and resolving ethical problems are rarely taught in medical schools. Persons whose education enables them to approach medical problems systematically and on the basis of objective data are now left with nothing more than personal intuition and common sense. Further, some physicians believe that no education or method could ever improve this situation. Ethical problems, they assert, are unique; they cannot be analyzed or generalized. Each person's decision, they affirm, is his alone, based on personal values. Finally, some physicians may feel no discomfort at all when confronted with ethical problems; either they simply refuse to acknowledge them or they reduce them to the technical dimensions of the case.

The authors recognize the physician's discomfort with difficult ethical issues. However, this book is written with the belief that such discomfort can, to some extent, be alleviated. We identify typical situations in which ethical problems arise and illustrate ways for thinking systematically about their ethical features. We structure these problems so that their features can be clearly discerned and openly discussed. We do not solve every problem, but we do offer counsel in the form of suggestions that are reasonable and practical from our point of view. At best these suggestions will meet wide acceptance; at worst they will give those who disagree something definite to argue against. We admit the final decision will be made in the privacy of conscience, but we believe conscientious decisions can be made only after reviewing considerations that others have thought relevant. Thus, we provide those considerations as completely, but as briefly, as we can.

This book presents an approach to clinical ethics for physicians who practice internal and general medicine. By clinical ethics, we mean the identification, analysis, and resolution of moral problems that arise in the care of a particular patient. These moral concerns are inseparable from the medical concerns about the correct diagnosis and treatment of the patient (Chapter 1). They will appear in light of the preferences patients express or do not express about their care and their future (Chapter 2). They will appear when certain sorts of futures are envisioned for that patient by others, such as physician and family (Chapter 3). They will be suggested by such matters as the costs of the patient's care and the availability of resources for proper care (Chapter 4).

In general, good clinical medicine is ethical medicine. Good clinical medicine consists in technical skill together with its sensitive application to the personal needs of the person asking for help in the care of his/her health. We believe clinical ethics is inextricably linked to the physician's primary task, deciding on and carrying out the best clinical care for a particular individual in a particular set of circumstances.

The practice of medicine is a meeting between two persons, one seeking help and the other offering it. That meeting differs greatly from an encounter with one's plumber, garage mechanic, or insurance agent. It is an encounter with life-and-death implications, which arouses deep psychological forces and engages one person, the patient, who is in distress and vulnerable, with another person, the physician, who is skilled and authoritative. Such a meeting imposes stringent moral demands on both parties; it requires trust, honesty, cooperation, competence, compassion. Today no one questions this view as an ideal, although achievement of the ideal is indeed difficult.

Even when physicians firmly adhere to the high moral standards that should govern the relationship between themselves and their patients, moments of "ethical indecision" will occur. In the course of deciding how best to care for a patient, the general moral maxims such as "above all, benefit the patient," "do no harm," "communicate honestly," or "do not let personal values prejudice medical decisions" may not always serve as adequate guides to conduct. Whether one maxim or another should apply may be unclear: Confidentiality, for example, may not be beneficial to a particular patient. The extent of a maxim's application may be unclear: Exactly how much information should be provided in an honest communication? These sorts of problems, rather than the general moral maxims of the patient–physician relationship, constitute the subject matter of clinical ethics. We try to show how these general and diverse maxims can be brought closer to the clinical situation in which a decision is to be made.

Philosophers and other philosophically minded readers may be troubled by the brevity of our considerations, which may strike them as superficial. We appreciate their complaint. However, this book is written not for philosophers but for physicians who are responsible for making clinical judgments about diagnosis and treatment for their patients. The authors judge that this audience needs a systematic approach for those decisions rather than a theory to elucidate (or obfuscate) the philosophy behind that approach. We are vividly aware that our concepts, our considerations, and the counsel we offer can be further analyzed and criticized in the light of ethical theory. We have drawn on those theories, yet we refrain from theoretical analysis or discursus. We refer our readers to the *Encyclopedia of Bioethics* (EB) and to our other bibliographical citations for the deeper and broader discussion of the issues we treat so briefly (EB: ETHICS; BIOETHICS).

This book also lacks several other elements that some readers might expect in a book entitled "ethics." It does not endeavor to reform systems or to urge those who participate in them to act more in accord with ideals. We do not question the need for reform of many features in medicine, from the training of its practitioners to the delivery of health care. However, this book is not devoted to those problems. It does not explore the need for reform or suggest how reform might be accomplished. Indeed, many of the problems it does discuss arise within and, probably, as a result of institutions, programs, and policies that are themselves unjust. Still, we confine our remarks to how one deals with the problem when it arises in the current system. One should work for reform in the future, but decisions must be made and actions taken by clinicians who work in the imperfect world of the present.

The authors are also aware that some religious traditions have highly developed medical ethics. We have not drawn on these traditions to formulate substantive positions. We have, on occasion, mentioned the more prominent positions of one or another religious tradition. We suggest that physicians who do adhere to a religious faith with an explicit ethic about medicine, such as

Roman Catholicism or Judaism, refer to the excellent books cited in the bibliography that express the doctrines of those faiths. (EB: ETHICS, THEOLOGICAL; PROTESTANTISM: JUDAISM; ROMAN CATHOLICISM.)

It should also be noted that, although legal matters are mentioned in this book, it is not a book on legal medicine. The brief discussion of legal matters is necessary because legal and ethical considerations are often mingled in clinical ethical decisions. However, anyone who needs legal advice should rely not on these pages but on the proper persons and sources.

PRESENTATION OF ETHICAL ASPECTS OF A CLINICAL CASE

Every good clinician has learned, from the first days of medical school, to "present" a patient in an organized fashion so that diagnostic and therapeutic possibilities can be systematically explored. Similarly, this book suggests a way to "present a patient" for an ethical decision: organizing and displaying the relevant data and questions in view of a practical *ethical* decision. This should help in arranging questions, gathering data, focusing on central points, excluding extraneous ones, and weighing evidence. It does not dictate conclusions. Conclusions must be drawn by the conscientious clinician after using the method to clarify and consolidate her thinking and feeling about a case.

The method for displaying the considerations involved in a clinical ethical decision consists of four general categories into which most of the considerations raised in any clinical case can be distributed. They are (1) Indications for Medical Intervention, (2) Patient Preferences, (3) Quality of Life, (4) External Factors. Each of these categories has a twofold significance. First, it can be filled up with the actual facts, opinions, and circumstances which persons involved in the particular case are likely to bring forth. Second, each category reflects certain major moral principles and moral values that have been considered important in the ethics of medicine and health care. Those acquainted with the philosophical literature might recognize the Principle of Beneficence Behind Indications for Medical Intervention, the Principle of Autonomy Behind Patient Preferences, and some form of Utilitarianism Behind Quality of Life and External Factors. Thus, by sorting out facts, opinions, and circumstances raised in the actual situation into categories that also can be viewed in light of an extensive body of ethical theory, it becomes possible to evaluate those facts, opinions, and circumstances in relation to each other. An ethical judgment, like a clinical judgment, follows from a perception of the various facts, opinions, and circumstances assessed for their ethical importance in the particular situation.

Assessing the importance of facts, opinions, and circumstances in the light of ethical categories is, of course, the most perplexing task. When facts, opinions, and circumstances are meshed with our ethical categories, we call them considerations. No ethical scales exist into which considerations can be poured until "importance" shows up on a precisely calibrated gauge. Still, rough measures can be made and are made in everyday life. In this book the rough measures are established by setting the four categories in order of priority. In the encounter between patient and physician (in the ideal situation), it is the physician's duty to recommend treatment that is medically indicated; it is the patient's right to accept or refuse those recommendations in the light of personal preferences. Thus, in the priority ordering, patient preferences are the weightiest ethical category in the physician-patient encounter. It is not so simple, of course: The ethical problems arise only when medical indications clearly point to a treatment that a patient refuses to authorize. Then questions are asked such as, "What is the purpose envisioned by this treatment choice? What is the patient's need? Is the patient really competent? Can the patient's need ever be so great as to override his preferences?" Questions of this sort will be answered by pointing to various facts and by offering opinions. These facts and opinions, in turn, will be assessed for their relative importance. This assessment may lead to the conclusion, in a particular case, that the order of priority has shifted. For example, decisions based on medical indications take priority when the patient is incompetent.

Some clinical situations exist in which the indications for treatment are questionable and the preferences of patients undiscernible. When that is so, questions about quality of life or about the importance of such "external factors" as costs or family burdens may be raised. In our ranking, neither quality-of-life choices that are not expressed as the patient's own preferences nor external factors have great ethical weight in clinical decisions. They move toward importance only as medical indications and patient preferences become, for various reasons explained in the text, less important. Our initial ranking of the order of ethical importance is (1) Patient Preferences, (2) Medical Indications, (3) Quality of Life, (4) External Factors. The manner in which this initial order is shifted in particular cases so that those lower in the scale move toward greater importance is explained in the text.

Finally, a word about language. We use several words over and over again. We speak of considerations as being "relevant," "important," and "decisive." These three words express our estimation of the place a consideration takes on our scale. "Relevant" simply means a consideration has some place in the deliberations about an ethical problem: It is not ruled out of court as "inadmissible evidence." To take a crude example, the obvious poverty of a person injured in an automobile accident is *not relevant* to a decision to provide help. If a consideration is "relevant," it will have various degrees of importance. Its greater or lesser significance can sometimes be seen intuitively; at other times it must be sought by analyzing carefully the various reasons offered for or against it. For example, it is not intuitively obvious whether the request of a patient who asks to be "put out of my misery" should or should not be honored. The importance of that preference must be judged by careful analysis of the arguments pro and con active euthanasia [3.3].* Finally, an "important" consideration may emerge as "decisive" when, after careful exploration of the implications and of other values, it appears to tip the scales in favor of a particular choice. A "decisive" consideration is one which, in view of all other relevant and important considerations, carries the greatest weight. Certainly, there will be many arguments about what counts as decisive, but we believe that in many clinical situations a large measure of agreement can be reached by thoughtful review of the relevant and important considerations.

We also use the terms "permissible" and "obligatory." An ac-

* Bracketed numbers within the body of the text refer the reader to appropriate sections elsewhere in the book. The first digit indicates the chapter in which the section is to be found.

tion is "permissible" when, after sufficient analysis, no "decisive" consideration emerges. "Important" considerations can be offered for alternatives, and the person faced with the choice thus may not be constrained to one or another of the alternatives. When a decisive consideration does emerge in favor of one alternative, we state that, in our view, that alternative is obligatory. Thus, we propose that it is permissible to remove from a respirator a person in the persistent vegetative state [3.2]. It is obligatory, we believe, to respect a competent patient's refusal of treatment (except in quite specific circumstances [2.5]).

HOW TO USE THIS BOOK

This book has four chapters entitled "Medical Indications," "Patient Preferences," "Quality of Life," and "External Factors." Each chapter addresses one of the principal areas where ethical questions arise. However, when these questions arise in actual clinical situations, they represent problems that cross boundaries between the subjects discussed in any single chapter. In order to comprehend these complex problems, the book has extensive cross-references. In addition, the contents are described in two ways: in a conventional Table of Contents (pp. xi–xii) and in a Locator (pp. xiii–xvii). The Locator is organized alphabetically by topic, and the topics are listed both under the terms of medical ethics, e.g., "passive euthanasia" and those terms more familiar to the clinician, e.g., "no code orders." The Locator lists all sections of the book where points relevant to a complete discussion can be found. Suppose you are faced with a particular problem, for example, a Jehovah's Witness refuses a blood transfusion. You can research this problem by looking at the Table of Contents for a heading that seems likely to treat the issue, e.g., Refusal of Treatment. Or you can check the Locator under any number of topics, e.g., Refusal of Treatment, Jehovah's Witnesses, Unusual Beliefs, Competence. The Locator entry will indicate the most extensive discussion of the problem by an underlined number and also show other sections that treat aspects of the problem. By glancing at each of these places, you should find all the relevant features of your case; you can display them, in your mind or for others, in order to assess their importance and to reach a well-reasoned and responsible decision.

Readers may wish to examine problems more deeply than they can in our text. References to articles in the *Encyclopedia of Bioethics* are noted in the text. At the end of the book, citations to a few books and articles are provided under the numbers that identify the passage in the text. These books and articles are a mixture of theoretical and practical discussions of the issues.

Our book is designed to be a useful guide for clinicians. It will describe many of the clinical ethical situations encountered in medical practice. It will provide a general approach that can be applied to many cases. And, finally, it will offer counsel about many specific ethical difficulties that clinicians are likely to encounter in the course of their practice.

Our success in achieving our goals will be measured by how useful and practical our handbook is for students, house officers, and practicing physicians. We hope clinicians and students will become more comfortable and confident in dealing with these difficult matters. If proper attention comes to be given to the ethical problems that arise in clinical decision-making, we will have achieved our purpose. Competent and confident physicians who are willing and able to deal with clinical ethical matters when they arise will provide the best care to patients.

BIBLIOGRAPHY

Callahan, D. Bioethics as a Discipline. *Hastings Center Report,* 1973, **1**(1):66.

Callahan, D. The Shattuck Lecture: Contemporary Medical Ethics. *N Engl J Med,* 1980, **302:**1228.

Cassell, E. J. Making and Escaping Moral Decisions. *Hastings Center Studies,* 1973, **1**(2):53.

Chapman, C. B. On the Definition and Teaching of the Medical Ethic. *N Engl J Med,* 1979, **301:**630.

Clouser, K. D. Medical Ethics: Some Uses, Abuses, and Limitations. *N Engl J Med* 1975, **293:**384.

Clouser, K. D. What Is Medical Ethics? *Ann Intern Med,* 1974, **80:**657.

Englehardt, H. T., Spicker, S. (eds.). *Philosophical Medical Ethics.* Dordrecht: D. Reidel, 1977.

Gustafson, J. M. The Contributions of Theology to Medical Ethics. *Perspectives in Biology and Medicine,* 1976, **19:**247.

Gustafson, J. M., Hauerwas, S. (eds.). Theology and Medical Ethics. *J Med Phil,* 1979, **4**.

Holder, A. *Medical Malpractice Law.* New York: John Wiley, 1975.

Ingelfinger, F. J. Arrogance. *N Engl J Med,* 1980, **303:**1507.

Jonsen, A. R., Can an Ethicist Be a Consultant? In Abernethy, 1980: 157.*

Jonsen, A. R., Hellegers, A. E. Conceptual Foundations for an Ethics of Medical Care. In Tancredi, L. (ed.), *Ethics of Health Care.* Washington, D.C.: Institute of Medicine, 1973. (In Reiser, Dyke, Curran, 1977, 129.)

Mitchell, B. Is a Moral Consensus in Medical Ethics Possible? *J Med Ethics,* **2:**18.

Pellegrino, E. Toward a Reconstruction of Medical Morality: The Primacy of the Act of Profession and the Fact of Illness. *J Med Phil,* 1979, **4:**32.

Pellegrino, E. *Humanism and the Physician.* Knoxville: University of Tennessee Press, 1979.

Rachels, J. Can Ethics Provide Answers? *Hastings Center Report,* 1980, **10**(3):32.

Siegler, M. A Legacy of Osler: Teaching Clinical Ethics at the Bedside. *JAMA,* 1978, **239:**951.

Siegler, M. Clinical Ethics and Clinical Medicine. *Arch Intern Med,* 1979, **139:**914.

Thompson, E. I. The Implications of Medical Ethics. *J Med Ethics,* 1976, **2:**75.

Twiss, S. The Problem of Moral Responsibility in Medicine. *J Med Phil,* 1977, **2:**376.

Veatch, R. M. From Cases to Rules: The Challenge in Contemporary Medical Ethics. In Abernethy, 1980: 48.

* Complete citations for abbreviated references appear at the end of the book (see General References).

1

INDICATIONS FOR MEDICAL INTERVENTION

1.0 This chapter discusses clinical judgment regarding the risks and benefits of diagnostic and therapeutic procedures insofar as these clinical judgments are related to ethical problems. It proposes three disease models, which represent types of medical problems commonly seen by the general physician. It then describes the sorts of ethical problems that might be associated with each of these models. It discusses in detail three ethical problems in which clinical judgment is particularly important: (1) the decision to terminate therapy for the patient no longer competent; (2) the decision not to resuscitate a patient in event of cardiorespiratory arrest; and (3) the criteria for determining that a patient has died.

The ethical principle underlying much of this chapter is the principle of "beneficence," the duty of assisting others in need and avoiding harm. This principle is expressed in the history of medicine by the Hippocratic maxim: Be of benefit and do no harm. (EB: Care; Therapeutic Relationship; Paternalism; Codes of Medical Ethics.)

1.1 RESPONSIBILITIES OF THE PHYSICIAN

The physician's central responsibility is to use medical expertise to respond to the patient's request for help in the care of his or her health by (1) diagnosing that patient's condition, (2) informing and educating the patient about the condition—including its prognosis if treated or untreated—and about the various possible treatment alternatives, (3) recommending the course of action that the physician considers the best medical approach for that individual's problem, and (4) carrying out those procedures —for example, monitoring, prescribing—that are required by the approach chosen by the patient (or, if the patient cannot choose due to incompetence, those suitable for the patient).

1.1.1 **Evaluation of Individual Patient.** In making a recommendation about medical care, the physician will evaluate the individual patient before him in terms of (1) the seriousness of the condition in an organic sense; (2) the seriousness of the condition in the patient's eyes; (3) the need for urgent action; (4) the possible therapeutic benefits; (5) the potential risks of the intervention; (6) alternative courses of action and inaction; (7) the physical, psychological, and social impact upon the patient of all options; (8) the ability of the patient to participate in his or her own care; and (9) all of these in light of the patient's self-understanding, self-diagnosis, fears, and hopes.

1.1.2 **Clinical Discretion.** The process by which a physician reaches the best clinical decision has been called clinical reasoning or clinical judgment. Essential to this process is discretion, the ability to discern relevant distinctions, to discard extraneous facts, to penetrate to the heart of the matter, and to make choices of one course of action as the best among many possible ones. That choice can be defended as "best" not in some absolute sense but because, given the available facts and their interpretation, judicious reflection suggests it fits the actual situation more adequately than other options available. Good choices about a patient's medical care require this clinical discretion; even more so do good ethical decisions.

Physicians must recognize that judgments about medical indications are not wholly and purely factual. These judgments are colored by values in many respects. Interpretation of data takes place within a complex context of assumptions. Clinical judgments reflect tacit inclinations about risk avoidance, skepticism about interventions, enthusiasm for innovation, fear of death, and many other personal values. Also, values that a physician may be loath to admit may bias outwardly "objective" judgments: anxiety regarding death and disability, disdain for certain kinds of persons or life styles, racial prejudices, repugnance for the aged or retarded. It is important to be aware of the subtle value aspects of objective medical judgments and to recognize that they may on occasion determine the clinical decision.

In a clinical ethical decision, discretion must comprehend a correct perception of the medical indications (Chapter 1), an appreciation of the patient's preferences (Chapter 2), an evaluation of the patient's quality of life (Chapter 3) and an awareness of external considerations, such as the role of the family, the costs of care, and so on (Chapter 4). Although these are treated in distinct chapters for pedagogical purposes, the physician must be able to draw them together, assess their importance, and reach a conclusion suited to a particular case. This is the act of clinical discretion. (EB: DECISION MAKING, MEDICAL.)

1.1.3 **Goals of Medical Intervention.** Medical indications are derived from the medical facts, together with available forms of treatment, which lead the physician to judge that some intervention may or may not be useful to the patient. Usually these indications point to quite immediate goals, e.g., treatment of a blood pressure of 180/115 with antihypertensive agents or prevention of symptoms of celiac sprue by prescribing a gluten-restricted diet.

However, behind these specific goals are the broader, more fundamental goals of medicine. There is no single goal of medicine. In the encounter between patient and physician many appropriate medical goals may be pursued simultaneously. These goals include:

1. Restoration of health
2. The relief of symptoms (including physical distress and psychological suffering)
3. The restoration of function or maintenance of compromised function

4. The saving or prolonging of life
5. The education and counseling of patients regarding their condition and its prognosis
6. Avoiding harm to the patient in the course of care

The simultaneous achievement of all these goals represents the most appropriate end for the particular encounter. This can be accomplished when a disease entity can be identified for which specific, curative therapy is available. In general, patients and physicians regard the identification and successful treatment of a curable condition to be the ideal endpoint of a medical encounter. (EB: THERAPEUTIC RELATIONSHIP.)

EXAMPLE. A twenty-four-year-old man has symptoms of severe headache and neck stiffness but has no other neurologic findings. The physician reaches a diagnosis of bacterial meningitis. In such a case, prompt diagnosis and treatment with a correct antibiotic is likely to achieve all the medical goals noted in 1.1.3.

1.1.4 **Partial Achievement of Medical Goals.** In many medical situations (in contrast to acute infectious illness, acute surgical problems such as appendicitis, or self-limited diseases which improve spontaneously) the achievement of a cure, a perfect outcome in which all the goals of medicine are realized, is less likely. For example, there is at present no definitive cure for many of the common chronic diseases of adulthood such as coronary artery disease, rheumatoid arthritis, chronic obstructive pulmonary disease, or diabetes mellitus. In dealing with these conditions, patients and physicians attempt to achieve partially some of the goals of medicine, such as relief of symptoms, patient education, retardation of functional impairment, prolongation of life, and maintenance of patient control and dignity. In these situations, in contrast to the curative model, tradeoffs frequently have to be made among competing goals.

EXAMPLE. A patient with chronic progressive respiratory deterioration continues to smoke cigarettes despite admonitions from the physician. A tradeoff may be occurring between prolongation of life and maintenance of function and the patient's wish to remain in control of his condition and to engage in behavior from which pleasure is derived.

1.1.5 **Realistic Understanding of the Goals of Treatment.** In particular cases this is essential to sound clinical discretion. It is equally essential to ethical deliberation in the process of clinical discretion. In a clinical case, ethical deliberation should begin with a clear and realistic evaluation of the goals of intervention for the patient under consideration. The assessment of which particular goals are *desired* from a medical encounter should be a determination made jointly by patient and physician after the patient has been informed by the physician as to which goals are *possible*. It is important to distinguish between the goals of medical intervention, to which this chapter is devoted, and the goals of the encounter between patient and physician, to which the other three chapters are also pertinent. In defining the goals of the encounter, the physician will consider:

(a) *The nature of the disease.* What goals are achievable for this particular patient who has this specific condition? Of course, any such determination in medicine must be expressed in probabilities rather than certainties. (This first factor will be discussed in considerable detail throughout the remainder of Chapter 1.)

(b) *The preferences of the patient.* What are the patient's goals in this medical encounter? In many instances, the patient's goals are indistinguishable from the physician's goals. However, it must be acknowledged that for personal, psychological, social, religious, or economic reasons, the patient's goals may differ from those of the physician. (Chapter 2 will discuss patients' preferences and how they influence medical action.)

(c) *The values of physicians and patients.* Although many physicians share with patients a common perspective on the ideal goals of medicine—the cure of illness—there may be less agreement between them on which of the partial goals of medicine is more or less desirable. This may be so particularly when that partial achievement leaves the patient with significant deficits, for example, continued life but with severe brain damage. If the patient is competent, these differing views can be discussed. When the patient is not competent, the values of the physician regarding "quality of life" must be carefully scrutinized. Further, it is also possible that physicians and patients may disagree over what goals are being sought and which goal is more desirable. (This difference in values is discussed in Chapter 3.)

(d) *Social, cultural, political, and economic realities.* Any goals sought by physicians and patients are pursued within a context of social, cultural, political, and economic realities. Availability of resources, the wealth or poverty of individuals and communities, religious and cultural beliefs, and so forth will facilitate the attainment of some goals and render others impossible. (These factors will be considered at length in Chapter 4.)

1.2 THREE GENERAL MODELS OF DISEASE AND TREATMENT

In this chapter we focus on the first important feature that determines physicians' actions, namely, the nature of the disease process. We begin our analysis of the goals and outcomes of treatment by examining three general models of disease/treatment situations.

1.2.1 **Three Models of Disease (ACURE, CARE, COPE) and Their Relationship to Clinical Ethical Decisions.** Physicians habitually approach medical problems by attempting to determine the indications for or against medical intervention. We suggest that they should approach ethical problems in the same manner. The first point in "presenting a patient" in view of an ethical problem should be a careful assessment of medical indications. However, that assessment will have to look beyond the probable immediate goals of any particular intervention (e.g., the likelihood that blood pressure will be raised by vasopressors or that lungs will be cleared by an antibiotic) toward the more fundamental goals of medicine [1.1.3]. In some situations medical indications will be very obvious, e.g., the patient is in diabetic ketoacedosis: All medical indications clearly favor immediate insulin administration and fluid repletion. In such cases the only sorts of ethical problems likely to arise would have to do with patient's preferences not to be treated, expressed previously or in a "living will," or the prospective quality of life of a particular patient (cf. Chapters 2 and 3). In other cases, the medical indications themselves may lie at the center of the problem, e.g., should heart and lung functions be artificially maintained for a patient in the terminal stages of cancer? Should infection or cardiac arrest be treated in such a patient? Here questions about the beneficial nature of results of medical intervention can be raised. It might be asked whether medical intervention is useful, whether medicine is achieving its goals.

Three models are presented to illustrate the relation between medical interventions and medical goals: (1) an acute, life-threatening disease, which we designate as ACURE; (2) a chronic, lethal disease, which we call CARE; and (3) a chronic, debilitating disease, COPE.

1.2.2 **The Uncertainties of Medicine.** Clinical medicine is "a science of uncertainty and an art of probability" (Osler). Experienced physicians appreciate that the most mature expression of the clinician's skill is the ability to make consistently good decisions when faced with uncertainty. In the following discussion concerning different disease models (which we have labeled ACURE, CARE, COPE), a series of terms such as *acute, chronic, critical, reversible,* and *easily treatable* are employed. These terms should be understood as probability statements rather than absolute designations. Nevertheless, more often than not clinicians would agree on whether a particular case represented, for example, an acute process, a chronic process, or an acute exacerbation of a chronic process.

1.3 THE FIRST MODEL: ACURE (Acute, Critical, Unexpected, Responsive, Easily Diagnosed and Treated)

CLINICAL EXAMPLE OF ACURE MODEL. A twenty-four-year-old university student comes to an emergency room with complaints of high fever, headache, and stiff neck. Physical examination suggests a diagnosis of meningitis. The student's mental status appears intact, and no focal neurological deficits are detected. The student gives consent for a spinal fluid examination, which confirms the diagnosis of meningitis. A gram stain of the spinal fluid reveals many gram positive diplococci suggestive of pneumococcal meningitis. The student is informed of the diagnosis and the physician recommends admission to the hospital for antibiotic treatment.

1.3.1 **The Relevant Features of the ACURE Model.** In ACURE cases the disease begins abruptly, is immediately life-threatening, is unanticipated, and is caused by factors beyond the patient's control. Further, diagnostic uncertainty is minimal; treatment is relatively easy, standardized, and effective; and without treatment the possibility of death or permanent disability is great. Each term in the ACURE model requires some description and explanation:

(a) *Acute.* Acute disease is contrasted with chronic disease. An acute disease is one which unfolds in a short time (minutes or hours or days, in contrast to months or years).

EXAMPLE. Respiratory failure from anaphylaxis is an acute illness whereas recurring bronchitis and obstructive pulmonary disease represent a chronic process.

(b) *Critical.* The word "critical" is a prognostic term specifying diseases that are immediately life-threatening (in contrast to slowly progressive diseases) or that will cause immediate, serious, and irreversible functional disabilities in addition to whatever symptoms they may cause.

EXAMPLE. Respiratory failure is a critical disease, while progressive respiratory insufficiency with functional impairment and chronic biochemical abnormalities represents a serious symptomatic illness that is not immediately critical.

(c) *Unexpected.* Unexpected diseases are those which are not anticipated by either the patient or the physician. They are contrasted with an inevitable crisis that will occur in the course of chronic or terminal diseases.

EXAMPLE. A patient who experiences a first anaphylactic reaction to penicillin, which results in respiratory failure has an unexpected disease. By contrast, an episode of acute respiratory decompensation that occurs in someone with severe, chronic underlying pulmonary disease would not be unexpected.

(d) *Reversible.* This concept designates the ability to alter the natural history of a disease by intervening with definitive, effective therapy (in contrast to palliative or symptomatic relief), thereby restoring the individual to the level of health and functioning enjoyed prior to the onset of this illness. *Terminal* illness is the opposite of reversible illness. Terminal illness may be acute or chronic; it is by definition *critical;* but also, by definition, specific therapy is not available to prevent functional deterioration or to save the patient's life. Palliative therapy to relieve symptoms or to prolong life is often available.

EXAMPLE. Respiratory failure resulting from an anaphylactic reaction to penicillin should be entirely reversible if the patient is treated quickly enough and adequately. By contrast, respiratory failure that results from lymphangitic dissemination of an untreatable neoplasm is not reversible, although palliative therapy may be available to temporarily relieve some symptoms.

(e) *Easily treated and diagnosed.* Some diseases are simple to diagnose and treat. In such conditions standardized, conventional, often "one-shot" therapy, such as an operation, short-term use of a respirator, or a course of medication (such as antibiotics) can eliminate the critical condition.

EXAMPLE. Ventilator support in respiratory failure from penicillin anaphylaxis should be contrasted with long-term treatment such as chronic ventilator therapy for end-stage pulmonary disease. The simple, easy treatments must be distinguished from long-term discomforting therapies such as cancer chemotherapy, burn management, and chronic renal dialysis, as well as from high-risk experimental therapy such as bone marrow transplantation and heart transplantation.

1.3.2 **Clinical Goals in the ACURE Model.** ACURE situations allow patients and physicians to achieve most of the traditional goals of the medical encounter, particularly curing disease, saving life, preserving function, relieving pain and suffering, and restoring health. Further, the medical indication for treatment, the wishes of the physician to treat, and the desire of the patient usually coincide. When this is so, the situation is medically and ethically unproblematical.

1.3.3 **Clinical Ethical Problems in ACURE Situations.** Even in seemingly straightforward situations such as the ACURE model described in 1.3, ethical problems may appear and may cause clinicians considerable difficulty. With reference to the case presented in 1.3, consider the ethical difficulties that might arise, given the following changes in the situation:

(a) The patient refuses to accept antibiotic treatment (as either an inpatient or an outpatient). The patient provides no reason for refusal. [Cf. 2.5.]

(b) After initially refusing therapy, the patient becomes lethargic and confused. The physician is concerned about treating a patient without obtaining informed consent. The physician has been led to believe that treating people without informed consent may constitute battery. [Cf. 2.3.]

(c) The patient refuses therapy, but the patient's family demands the physician treat the patient. [Cf. 4.2.]

(d) The patient presented in 1.3.1 was known to suffer from a life-threatening underlying disease such as uncontrolled acute myeloblastic leukemia, which had failed to respond to several previous chemotherapy regimens. [Cf. 1.4.3–1.6.4.]

(e) The patient consented to be admitted and treated. The admitting physician tried to place the patient in the neurology/neurosurgery intensive care unit (ICU), but no beds were available in the unit. The admitting physician demanded that the resident on duty in the ICU transfer an elderly stroke victim in order to make room for the student with meningitis. [Cf. 4.5–4.5.4.]

COMMENT. Each of the modifications in 1.3.3 introduces an ethical quandary into a clinical situation otherwise simple and unproblematical. The practicing physician is now called upon to make a series of judgments that are not precisely "technical," although they are surely "clinical" decisions. How should these situations be handled? The clinician's first response to any ethical problem like those posed above should be to locate the patient clearly within the ACURE model in terms of the nature of the disease, the kinds of intervention possible, and the attainable goals.

1.4 THE SECOND MODEL: CARE (Critical, Active, Recalcitrant, Eventual)

Clinical Example of CARE Model. A thirty-four-year-old man with a fifteen-year history of confirmed multiple sclerosis has had several flareups of his illness, which have left him severely disabled. His initial attack consisted of numbness and weakness of his right leg and decreased visual acuity in the left eye. These signs resolved, but two years later he developed spasticity and weakness in his left leg. Although he was told his diagnosis and although his physician attempted on several occasions to explain the nature and course of multiple sclerosis, the patient refused to participate in such discussions. He specifically requested the physician not to inform him of his prognosis.

During the past twelve years the patient has experienced episodic but progressive physical deterioration. He developed severe spasticity in his leg. He used two canes and later a walker to ambulate but is currently confined to a wheelchair. His visual acuity has declined and he is now functionally blind in one eye and almost blind in the other. He has been unable to get a penile erection and last engaged in sexual activities six years ago. Five years ago he developed bladder dysfunction and has required an indwelling Foley catheter for the past three years. In recent years, he has required repeated admissions for the management of urinary tract problems associated with his atonic bladder and indwelling Foley catheter, and on one occasion he was treated for documented gram-negative septicemia and pyelonephritis. He has also experienced difficulty controlling his oral secretions and has had two episodes of pneumonia requiring hospitalization in recent years. He has deep decubitus ulcers and probable chronic osteomyelitis. His mental status is difficult to evaluate. He is profoundly depressed, and some observers think the depression is associated with the early development of dementia.

1.4.1 **Clinical Features of the CARE Model.** The CARE model describes patients who suffer from a critical disease that has active, progressive, and deleterious effects. Such conditions are often chronic, but the CARE model also describes acute incurable illness. Such chronic and acute diseases are recalcitrant to any treatment that can either cure the disease or reverse its deleterious effects (although optimal medical care may retard such effects or alleviate symptoms). Further, the probable direct outcome from the disease or its medical complications is the death of the patient. In chronic CARE situations, the patient is usually informed and knowledgeable about the disease and its likely course. Each term in the CARE model requires description and explanation:

(a) *Critical.* In 1.3.1b, we defined a critical disease as one that was immediately life-threatening or caused immediate, serious, and irreversible functional disabilities. The CARE model also describes patients who suffer from a critical disease with active, progressive, and deleterious effects. CARE situations include patients with diseases such as multiple sclerosis (described above in 1.4), metastatic cancer, or chronic cardiac, pulmonary, or hepatic failure.

The CARE model includes two forms of critical illness: (1) that which occurs as an acute exacerbation of a chronic disease and (2) that which occurs as the end-stage of a chronic, progressive disease. In contrast to ACURE diseases, critical illness that develops in the CARE model is usually not unexpected but represents anticipated progression of the underlying disease.

> EXAMPLE. The case of Mr. CARE [1.4] represents an example of acute, critical disease (a life-threatening infection) superimposed on the chronic condition of multiple sclerosis. However, Mr. CARE's entire course of frequent and multiple infections, which are themselves not preventable by any medical or social intervention, suggests that his entire disease state has now reached the *critical* stage. One of these multiple episodes of infection will probably prove fatal. Thus his underlying disease can be described as having reached a critical stage, and also certain acute exacerbations of the underlying disease may themselves be critical.

(b) *Active.* Many diseases are chronic and only slowly progressive. At some point, most chronic conditions enter a stage of activity in which the disease progresses rapidly and causes symptoms, functional impairment, and eventual death. In contrast to the COPE model [1.9], CARE describes diseases that have entered this stage of active progression. CARE can also be used to describe certain illness (for example, extensive burns, massive intracerebral hemorrhage, or carcinomatosis). These are invariably fatal, but they present not as chronic conditions but as acute, incurable diseases.

EXAMPLE. A patient with postnecrotic cirrhosis has had ascites and esophageal varices for several years. Over the course of several months, the patient develops hepatic encephalopathy, a decrease in hepatic synthetic function with prothrombin time prolongation (unresponsive to parenteral vitamin K therapy), progressive and uncontrollable ascites, and several episodes of acute esophageal bleeding. This patient's chronic progressive disease has entered the *active* phase and the disease has shifted from one managed in the COPE model to one that represents the CARE model.

(c) *Recalcitrant and eventual.* The CARE model refers to disease processes that are not entirely reversible. Examples of such conditions include multiple sclerosis, untreatable metastatic malignancies, and the late stages of pulmonary, cardiac, or hepatic failure. At the CARE stage, the treatment of such conditions does not consist of simple, "one-shot" therapy. However, individual acute problems may respond to simple interventions such as antibiotics for an infectious complication. If therapy is available for the underlying CARE problem, it tends to be long-term and difficult, such as cancer chemotherapy or renal dialysis, or even experimental, such as cardiac or bone marrow transplantation.

EXAMPLE. The multiple sclerosis patient described in 1.4 will be subject to repeated infections from multiple sources—lungs, bladder, skin, and bone. Even if his physicians were, for example, to treat his osteomyelitis with antibiotics and surgery, and his decubitus ulcers with skin grafts, this therapy would improve his situation only slightly. Further, they would subject the patient to the risks of general anesthesia needed to perform these several operative procedures. The patient's disease is now not only active but also recalcitrant.

Death will eventually occur, and in this instance the term eventual is used to describe a grim prognosis measured in months or weeks rather than in years. [Cf. 1.6.1.b]

1.4.2 **Clinical Goals in CARE Model.** In contrast to the ACURE model in which most of the goals of medicine are achievable [1.1.3], in the CARE model physicians and patients must lower their clinical expectations [1.1.4]. Thus, in CARE situations cure or restoration of function may not be possible, and appropriate goals of intervention might include prolongation of life, relief of pain and suffering, maximal preservation of limited function, and enhancement of the patient's dignity and sense of control regarding his/her disease and life.

1.4.3 **The CARE Model and Some Clinical Ethical Problems.** As noted in section 1.2.1, the physician's first response to a patient's problem should be framed in the context of an assessment of the indications for medical intervention. *In this regard, the assignment of the patient to the CARE rather than ACURE model is an important step in moving toward clinical-ethical decision*. This assignment is an act of clinical discretion, which requires the establishment of a diagnosis, prognosis, and therapeutic plan. For the physician these factors determine which medical goals are potentially achievable in the clinical encounter.

In general, CARE patients who are capable of expressing a choice or who have expressed and made known their wishes in the past are more likely to influence the treatment they receive than ACURE patients. At either end of the spectrum of CARE cases—asymptomatic patients or those who are terminally ill—the preferences of the patient should be decisive in determining how much and what kind of treatment such patients receive. (Cf. Chapter 2.)

However, the CARE model will often present situations in which the patient's preferences cannot be directly expressed. This may take place in the advanced stages of the chronic disease, when the patient's ability to reason and/or communicate may be disrupted by the disease or its complications [cf. 2.2]. When this takes place, the judgment of the physician that medical treatment is no longer useful may become the decisive ethical consideration. "No longer useful" in this context means that medical intervention is judged not likely to attain any of the goals of medicine or that it may attain one or another of those goals which, in the absence of others, is not of independent and overriding importance. [Cf. 1.1.3–1.1.5.;1.5.]

1.4.4 Consideration of Certain Developments of the CARE Case Presented in 1.4

(a) *Decision to withdraw life support.* Mr. CARE, now in the advanced stages of multiple sclerosis and suffering many complications, is in the ICU on a respirator. He is sinking rapidly. Vital signs are BP 60/40 on dopamine; pO_2 30 on PEEP 10 mm. Should the respirator be turned off? [1.5.]

(b) *Decision not to intubate.* Mr. CARE, still living in his home, lapses into coma. He is brought to the hospital and is admitted for treatment of urinary tract infection, gram-negative septicemia, shock, and the adult respiratory distress syndrome. Therapy is begun immediately with fluids, antibiotics, and pressor agents, but the patient's physician hesitated before intubating him and placing him on a respirator [3.2].

(c) *Orders not to resuscitate.* Mr. CARE is placed on a respirator. He recovers from the episode of gram-negative septicemia and shock. However, probably as a result of cerebral anoxia, his mental status deteriorated further and he now has a profound dementia. After being transferred from the ICU to a regular nursing unit, his physician thinks that he should be made a "no-code" case [Cf. 1.6.]

(d) *Irreversible coma/brain death.* Mr. CARE experiences a respiratory arrest on the way to the emergency room and probably suffers ten minutes of cerebral anoxia before adequate ventilation is reestablished. The patient is admitted to the ICU on a respirator. The patient has been comatose since admission. Doll's eyes, corneal reflexes, and pupillary reflexes are absent. Two EEGs show slow fluctuations with no defined rhythm. The nurses report some possible facial movements. A consulting neurologist believes the patient meets brain death criteria. One week later, despite recovery from gram-negative septicemia, the patient remains in deep coma. Physicians wonder how aggressively they should treat this patient with adult respiratory distress syndrome and whether it would be "right" to treat a new infection if it were to develop [1.7].

(e) *"Living will."* On admission, this patient's attorney contacts the physicians and informs them that the patient had executed a "living will" five years earlier and had updated it one year before. In this document the patient stated that, if a situation arose in which he was no longer able to speak or make decisions for himself, he absolutely did not want to be placed on a respirator, an "artificial breathing device" [2.6].

Situations (a), (b), (c), (d) are ethical problems typical of the CARE model. They will be discussed at length in the following sections. Situation (e), "the living will," will be discussed in Chapter 2, "Patient Preferences." Situations similar to (a), (b), and (c) that involve quality of life issues will be treated again in Chapter 3.

1.5 DECISIONS TO TERMINATE OR WITHHOLD INTERVENTION AS MEDICALLY INEFFICACIOUS

In 1.4.4 (a) and (b) Mr. CARE's situation is critical. The physician wonders about the efficacy of medical intervention: in (a) the continued use of the respirator, in (b) intubation and initiation of respirator support. Of course, the respirator will be efficacious in a certain sense, namely, gas exchange, compromised by ARDS, will be improved. This attains, in partial fashion, several of the goals of medicine: compromised function of several essential organ systems is maintained and, as a result, life is prolonged, at least for a time. However, the physician's doubts about efficacy are of a more fundamental nature: Given the presence of a lethal disease in its final stages and radical damage to multiple systems, none of medicine's other important goals will be attained. The patient certainly will not be restored to health; pain and symptoms will not be alleviated; compromised functions will not be restored or improved, but at best substituted for by mechanical means. Will further intervention be useful or efficacious in the larger sense?

(a) In 1.4.4(a), given the patient's vital signs, the patient appears to be close to death, whether or not the respirator is continued.

No medical intervention will reverse this course. If it does retard the course, clinical experience suggests it will be for several hours at best. It is ethically permissible to turn off the respirator.

(b) Considering the complexity of this patient's situation in 1.4.4(b), the probabilities of his recovery from sepsis and adult respiratory distress syndrome are low to the vanishing point. Although return to adequate lung function is remotely possible, even if this were accomplished, clinical experience with similar patients suggests this patient is entering the terminal phase of his illness. His survival, under the best of circumstances, will probably be no more than several weeks. The patient is not likely to emerge from his comatose condition. Medical intervention, while capable of prolonging life briefly and supporting compromised function, also prolongs the terminal stage of this patient's dying. Given this ambivalent attainment of medical goals, it is ethically permissible not to intubate.

COMMENT. A judgment about the inefficacy of treatment is the most obvious ethical justification for a decision to terminate or withhold medical intervention. There is no moral obligation to perform useless or futile actions. Thus, if none of the goals of treatment is attainable, that treatment need not be initiated or continued. In principle, all this seems clear; in practice, its application is difficult. First, many interventions are useful in the short run, e.g., Mr. CARE's urinary tract infection could very proably be cleared up. It is difficult to distinguish long-run from short-run efficacy. Second, one or another of the medical goals will probably be attained, e.g., prolongation of life, maintenance of function. Can we or should we rank them in importance? Third (and often very prominent in the clinical setting), there is frequently uncertainty about efficacy. It is difficult to know how long one must try some intervention before judging it inefficacious. It might also be difficult to judge whether another, yet untried, intervention might succeed when others have failed.

COUNSEL. (a) With regard to short-run and long-run efficacy, we advise that the distinction be explicitly and carefully made. In clinical settings there is a tendency to concentrate on short-run efficacy and to persist in interventions that have specific and likely results rather than to view the larger picture. For example, in 1.4.4(b), an ACURE situation is superimposed upon a CARE situation in its advanced stages. The ready therapies appropriate to ACURE should not be allowed to disguise the underlying and uncorrectable lethal process. Thus, in ethical discussion about patients of this sort, one must distinguish explicitly between long-run efficacy and short-run efficacy.

(b) With regard to the priority in importance of medical goals, we take the position that no general ranking of these goals is possible: Various goals are suited to various situations, e.g., restoration of health is a suitable goal for an ACURE situation; it is not an achievable goal for CARE or COPE. Relief from symptoms and stabilization of compromised function are suitable goals for CARE and COPE, *However, we do take the position that attainment of the single goal of prolonging life when progressive and critical deterioration of major systems seems to be leading to inevitable death is not an independent and overriding goal of medicine*. In the cases cited above, this seems to be the only goal in view. We consider that it alone is not sufficient to impose on the physician a moral obligation to continue intervention. Further discussion of this matter will be found in Chapter 3.

(c) With regard to uncertainty about efficacy, we suggest the following:

(i) Make a reasonable effort to dispel factual uncertainty about the probability of successful treatment by a literature search or by appropriate consultations.

(ii) Assess the evidence, from literature and from clinical experience, and reach a conclusion of reasonable certainty, that is, a judgment that reflects the weight of available evidence. Absolute certainty is neither possible nor necessary in judgments of this kind.

(iii) Distinguish doubt about efficacy from personal trepidation or hesitation in the face of so crucial a decision. The sensitive practitioner is bound to experience some trepidation. Also, distinguish doubt about efficacy from doubt about the ethical propriety of the act. We maintain that doubt about ethical propriety is dispelled by a reasonable judgment that further intervention is not useful in attaining the important goals of medicine. This judgment justifies the ethical propriety of the act in this case.

(iv) Recognize that procrastination, after the data are in, is itself a decision with ethical implications.

(v) If genuine doubt about efficacy remains, continue to treat. Significant evidence that a good chance remains to attain important goals of medicine makes intervention obligatory until time changes the picture.

NOTE. We have, in this entire discussion, presumed that no expression of the patient's preferences is available. If there were such expression, it must, of course, be taken into consideration. Patient preferences, indeed, may be the decisive consideration, either to continue or to stop treatment. The scope of this consideration is discussed in Chapter 2.

1.5.1 **"Passive Euthanasia."** We do not encourage the use of the phrase "passive euthanasia." It is conceptually unclear and leads to confusion. However, if used at all, the situations described in 1.5 seem closely to approximate the meaning intended by most authors. In these cases the ethical "passivity" consists not in the nonperformance of some physical act (the "omission" often spoken of in discussion of these cases). Certainly, in 1.4.4(a), the physician turns off the respirator (an act of commission). Rather, the passivity consists in standing by "passively" while allowing nature to take its course toward death; it is ethically permissible to stand by in this manner because there is no "active" duty to treat when treatment is judged useless or of minimal utility, that is, when it will attain only that goal which is not of overriding and independent importance, prolonging organic life. [On euthanasia, see 3.3–3.3.5.]

The principal religious denominations appear to accept this position. It is taught explicitly by the Roman Catholic Church [2.6.1]. While many Jewish teachers also accept it, strict Orthodox Judaism appears to be opposed. (EB: DEATH, WESTERN RELIGIOUS THOUGHT; DEATH AND DYING, ETHICAL VIEWS; JUDAISM; RELIGIOUS DIRECTIVES IN MEDICAL ETHICS.)

1.5.2 **Legal Liability.** A decision taken in accord with the above consideration appears to be free of legal liability. Even though a person dies as the result of the action or inaction of another who is responsible for the care of that person (thus, theoretically, a homicide is committed), the duty of that responsible person to provide care is terminated by the judgment of futility or uselessness of continuing. Legal liability, civil or criminal, could arise only when there is legitimate dispute about the facts of the case. Nevertheless, even in situations where futility of intervention is clear and no other legal issues are relevant, physicians may fear legal liability. They hesitate to decide or to record their decision and the reasons for it. We suggest that careful decision, consultation, and clear records are the best protection from liability.

1.6 ORDERS NOT TO RESUSCITATE (NO-CODE ORDERS)

In 1.4.4(c) Mr. CARE has recovered from the episode of gram-negative septicemia and from shock. His mental status has deteriorated and he is now profoundly demented. He is transferred from ICU to the ward, and a "no-code" order is suggested by the house officer.

Orders not to resuscitate or "no-code" refer to orders given by the attending physician or by the house officers that, if a particular patient suffers cardiac or respiratory arrest, cardiopulmonary resuscitation should not be attempted. As a result, the patient almost inevitably will die immediately. Indeed, it can be thought that the patient *had died,* due to cardiac arrest, and is being revivified (the French use the term "reanimation"). *The ethical grounds for such an order should be the sound medical judgment that the patient's death from primary disease is imminent and that further treatment for the primary disease is futile.* The distinction between this decision and the decision to terminate or withhold therapy is that (a) the patient is now in a relatively stable state, (b) death from the primary disease is anticipated very quickly, and (c) cardiac or respiratory failure is anticipated. [Cf. 3.2.]

Cardiopulmonary resuscitation (CPR) is a relatively new emergency medical technique that was developed to prevent sudden and unexpected death in the life-threatening situation of cardiopulmonary arrest. The existence of a medical technique or technology does not mandate its use in every case. It is the responsibility of the physician to decide which patients should be treated with which medical techniques, and the indications and contraindications to CPR should be examined in this context.

1.6.1 **Indications and Contraindications for CPR.** All persons who experience unexpected cardiopulmonary arrest for any known or unknown cause and who are not known to be terminally and irreversibly ill should be resuscitated. Most hospitals have a policy that all patients are "coded" unless there is a written order to the contrary. Age, mental disease, mental retardation, and chronic disease capable of being treated or palliated should not be grounds for withholding CPR unless special circumstances are present. The appropriate medical circumstances are presented in the following section. Other special circumstances are discussed in Chapter 3.

Standards for CPR, issued by the National Conference on CPR, state:

> The purpose of cardiopulmonary resuscitation is the prevention of sudden, unexpected death. Cardiopulmonary resuscitation is not indicated in certain situations, such as in cases of terminal, irreversible illness where death is not unexpected. . . . It has even been suggested that resuscitation in these circumstances may represent a positive violation of the individual's right to die with dignity. [*Standards and Guidelines for Cardiopulmonary Resuscitation* (*CPR*) *and Emergency Cardiac Care* (*ECC*). *JAMA* 1980; 244:453.]

COMMENTS. (a) *Terminal, irreversible illness, and imminent death.* CPR is not sound medical practice in the case of cardiopulmonary arrest that occurs as the anticipated end of a terminal illness. CPR should not be used on patients who are likely to succumb to their basic disease in a short time, on patients who are dying and suffering from intractable pain, or on patients who are irreversibly comatose.

(b) *Imminence of death.* One of the central concepts in deliberating about the ethical propriety of withholding CPR is the imminence of death. The question is often asked, "How imminent? How long before death is expected in the ordinary course of this disease?'' There is no precise answer in general or in the particular case. We must heed the words of Aristotle in the first book of his *Ethics:* ''Our discussion will be adequate if it has as much clearness as the subject matter admits of, for precision is not to be sought for alike in all discussions.'' In this vein, several comments on the notion of imminent death can be offered.

(i) Some have suggested that CPR policies be written to include a definite time for ''imminent death,'' such as two weeks. Presumably, this period of time would be estimated on the basis of clinical experience with patients suffering similar diseases. This ''seems more exact than the subject matter admits of,'' as well as improbable in light of the quite different courses of patients. A very experienced practitioner may be able to estimate the expected time span of a patient with a terminal illness, but it is unlikely that this prognostication can be generalized.

(ii) The word ''imminence'' not only means ''near or close in time''; it is etymologically derived from ''threatening, menacing.'' Thus, even though the time element may not be exact, the perception, by physicians, nurses, family, even the patient, if capable, that the end is menacingly near is important. All humans, of course, live under threat of death but, mercifully, we do not perceive its imminence at most times. When we do, a variety of factors warn of its arrival, many of which are clinically evident. Thus, imminent death should mean not only a short time, in terms of a few days or weeks, but also the perception of the menace of death's invasion.

(iii) The imminence of death also implies that, if resuscitated, the time remaining to the patient will be filled with pain, distress, further deterioration, and another critical moment (from which, in some institutions, the patient will again be rescued). It is this prospect which refraining from CPR is intended to avoid. If the time remaining is short, the ethical justification for refraining is based upon the futility of medical treatment: The patient is resuscitated only to die. If the remaining time is estimated to be longer, e.g., more than a month, the considerations relevant to quality of life should be reviewed (Chapter 3).

(iv) It should not be forgotten that the patient who suffers cardiac arrest is, at least in one sense, dead. Cardiopulmonary resuscitation, then, brings back to life by restoring heartbeat. Thus, if the patient is imminently dying of a lethal process, bringing back to life would be the ultimate in futility.

COUNSEL. (a) *Terminal and irreversible conditions.* CPR should be withheld from patients of the following sort who are in critical condition: patients with severe chronic disease such as cancer of the pancreas that has metastasized despite surgery and chemotherapy; patients with a progressive neurological condition such as Jacob-Creutzfeld disease; and patients with end-stage pulmonary, cardiac, or hepatic disease that has not responded to appropriate treatment.

Similarly, patients with these acute, seemingly irreversible diseases should probably not receive CPR: myocardial infarction with cardiogenic shock unresponsive to appropriate treatment, acute viral or bacterial pneumonias with unresponsive adult respiratory distress syndrome, massive intracerebral hemorrhage, or acute liver failure unresponsive to aggressive treatment. Often, CPR is not indicated in patients who have been treated vigorously for an acute problem for weeks in an ICU and whose state deteriorates and terminates in a cardiac arrest. If the vigorous therapy in the intensive care setting has not been successful, it is unlikely that a final, *pro forma* pounding on the chest or administration of one or several electrical shocks will reverse the progressive downhill course. The principal determinant of success in CPR relates to the patient's underlying disease. Thus, in such instances, even if CPR is temporarily successful, the patient is likely to arrest again unless some unexpected change occurs in the patient's underlying disease.

(b) *Uncertain situations.* There are many conditions in which physicians cannot be reasonably certain that a disease is terminal and irreversible. Many kinds of trauma, such as extensive burns, which in previous times would have been invariably fatal, can now be treated successfully. Further, a variety of life-threatening infectious illnesses, tumors (such as leukemias, lymphomas, and some carcinomas), and profound physiological derangements (such as the adult respiratory stress syndrome) may often be managed successfully. In the face of medical uncertainty, the presumptive obligation of the physician is to treat and to preserve the patient's life. Therefore, such patients usually should be candidates for CPR.

1.6.2 Who Makes the Decisions for CPR?

(a) *The physician.* In general, physicians must decide in view of the medical indications whether or not a patient is a candidate for CPR, i.e., whether a resuscitation effort is possible and appropriate. Although various guidelines have been published, none of them substitutes for clinical discretion. When the physician determines that a patient is terminally and irreversibly ill and that no additional course of therapy (or likely medical advance) offers any reasonable expectation of remission from the terminal condition, it is appropriate to write an order not to perform CPR on the patient.

(b) *The patient.* If the patient is competent, the patient may request that CPR not be performed. This request should be honored, if it is in accord with medical indications, (1.6.1). If it is not in accord with medical indications, considerations about refusal of treatment are relevant [2.5].

(c) If physicians decide the patient is not an appropriate candidate for CPR and the patient is mentally competent, the patient's permission not to resuscitate should be sought. Should the patient refuse, only the presence of decisive considerations regarding external factors (e.g., 4.4) should override the patient's preference. The patient's family should be informed, although their permission is not necessary either ethically or legally unless the patient is a minor or they have been declared legal guardians. The discussion with the patient and family should be summarized in the progress notes. It is unnecessary, offensive, and probably legally meaningless to ask the patient to sign some sort of "release" (see Chapters 2 and 4).

1.6.3 **Documentation of the Order.** Physicians should document the decision for an order not to resuscitate and should specify the reason for this decision. The documentation in the progress notes should include the medical fact and opinion underlying the order and a summary of discussion with patient, consultant staff, and family. Dissenting views also should be noted. The physician should then write an order stating the extent and duration of the decision in the order section of the chart. Everyone concerned with the care of the patient should be informed of the order not to resuscitate. Legal advice now favors an explicit record of this order and its reasons. Naturally, the order should be reviewed at regular intervals in view of the condition of the patient and should be changed when the condition of the patient warrants it.

1.6.4 **Interventions Other than CPR.** Orders not to resuscitate have been limited to refraining from CPR. In general, they should not be understood to apply to other interventions, such as refraining from the use of antibiotics, feeding or hyperalimentation, hydration, and other measures to provide comfort to the patient. The reason for this appears to be that cardiac arrest promises a swift and painless death to one who otherwise is certain to die more slowly and with greater discomfort. Refraining from other interventions may not have the same effect.

EXAMPLE. Karen Ann Quinlan was removed from the respirator when it was decided she would not return to "a cognitive and sapient state." She then began to breathe spontaneously. The question was raised whether a no-code order should be written, then whether infections should be treated and feedings continued. It was determined to write a no-code order and not to treat infections, but to continue feeding and hydration.

COMMENT. When it has been decided to retreat from more aggressive therapeutic efforts, physicians seem inclined to discontinue various interventions in a certain order. Roughly speaking, this order seems to be as follows: the withdrawal of experimental therapy such as extracorporeal membrane oxygenator or cardiac assist balloon pump; the decision not to perform CPR; the discontinuation of breathing support such as respirator; the discontinuation of agents that artificially maintain blood pressure and cardiac output; the decision not to intervene in the face of infections with antibiotic treatment; the decision to discontinue unusual forms of alimentation such as tube feeding or parenteral hyperalimentation; and finally the decision to reduce intravenous fluids to a maintenance or even, at times, a below-maintenance level.

In recent years new technological developments in feeding techniques and hydration, including intravenous therapy, enteral alimentation (through feeding tubes), and parenteral hyperalimentation through central venous catheters, have required an assessment of the appropriate use of these interventions. Physicians may come to view feeding and hydration technology as similar to respirators and artificial hearts. Irreversibly dying patients are now sometimes placed on a "TKO" status, i.e., intravenous catheters are used only "to keep open" and not to hydrate even at levels necessary to maintain bodily functions.

This stepwise retreat may appear illogical to some. They might assert that, once the imminence of death is acknowledged, efforts to forestall death should cease entirely. However, it is not so simple. First, recognition of the imminence and inevitability of death often dawns slowly. Second, the physician's investment of effort often breeds reluctance to admit defeat. Third, deep human sentiments about fighting death or providing nourishment lead to apparently illogical efforts to clear up infections or continue alimentation. Finally, physicians frequently are activists who are driven to "do something."

COUNSEL. (a) Decisions to withdraw or withhold specific interventions should be based upon the recognition of the progressively lessening achievability of medical goals. Above all, it should reflect the deliberate decision to change from goals that are curative to forms of care that provide comfort for the dying person. In a most important sense, the dying person is no longer a patient: "Once it has been determined that no further efforts will reverse the dying process, medical treatment is no longer in order. The dying person—no longer a patient—has the right to such comforts and easements as medicine provides, but he has neither the right to demand nor the duty to accept medical treatment." (Siegler and Osmond, 1979, p. 183.) Therefore, stepwise retreat should move from therapeutic interventions to comforting interventions.

(b) Some comforting interventions also have the effect of prolonging life, e.g., feeding and hydration. Recognition of the imminence of death does not impose an *obligation* on the physician to cease all life-prolonging methods; it *permits* the physician to turn from therapy to comforting methods.

(c) It is important that physicians make clear to all concerned the steps to be taken and the reasons for them.

1.7 BRAIN DEATH

In 1.4.4(d), the question was raised whether the patient was "brain dead." This term, introduced into clinical medicine during the last decade, causes much confusion. It is used most properly to describe a patient whose heart and lungs are being activated by a respirator but whose respiratory centers in the brain stem are destroyed. Thus, if removed from the respirator, the person would not resume spontaneous breathing. The person is "dead" in the sense of lacking the intrinsic, self-limiting capacity to sustain the most fundamental organic functions in an integrated manner. The language of the model legal statute regarding brain death expresses this by stating:

> An individual who has sustained either (1) irreversible cessation of circulatory and respiratory function, or (2) irreversible cessation of all functions of the entire brain, including the brain stem, is dead. A determination of death must be made in accordance with accepted medical standards. [President's Commission for Study of Ethical Problems in Medicine and in Biomedical and Behavioral Research; EB: DEATH, DEFINITION AND DETERMINATION OF.]

Also, the person is dead in the sense that the physical center of personal identity, the brain, is no longer functioning. However, since this also applies to persistent vegetative state, where it has further implications, it is discussed below and at 3.2.

1.7.1 **"Persistent Vegetative State."** Brain death, in the proper sense expressed above, should not be confused with the situation in which a person shows no evidence of cortical functioning, but continues to have sustained capacity for spontaneous breathing and heartbeat. This state can be called "cortical" or "cerebral" death or, more precisely, "persistent vegetative state." (Cf. American Neurological Association Criteria, ANA Transactions 102:172, 1977.)

1.7.2 **Differentiation of "Brain Death" and "Persistent Vegetative State."** The clinical signs differentiating "brain death" and "persistent vegetative state" are listed in Table I.

Table I. CLINICAL SIGNS*

Brain Death	*Persistent Vegetative State*
	Definition
Irreversible cessation of *all* functions of the brain	Irreversible cessation of *cognitive* (higher cortical) functions of the brain
	Autopsy Studies
Destruction of the entire brain (cerebral hemispheres and brain stem)	Extensive destruction of the cerebral cortex (neocortex)
	Sequence of Events
1. Primary insult 2. Development of cerebral edema, increased intracranial pressure 3. Intracranial pressure exceeds systolic blood pressure 4. *Permanent* loss of brain blood flow 5. Irreversible cessation of all brain functions	1. Systemic hypotension or hypoxia 2. Decreased brain blood flow or oxygen (transient) 3. Infarction of neocortex, ischemia of brain stem. (total ischemia or hypoxia: 4–6 minutes—destruction of neocortex; 15–20 minutes—destruction of entire brain) 4. Irreversible cessation of cognitive functions
	Clinical Examination
Coma (total unarousal, deepest possible coma) No movements, voluntary or involuntary (except spinal segmental reflexes) No brain stem reflexes (apnea, fixed pupils)	Awake, but unaware (profound dementia, not coma) No conscious interaction with the environment Eyes open; sleep-wake cycles Visual tracking movements Facial grimacing, yawning Spontaneous, involuntary movements Intact brain stem reflexes
	Treatment
Total respirator support Intensive medical management to maintain heart-lung preparation	Respirator dependent for usually a few days to a few weeks Management of medical complications (primarily pulmonary, infectious)

Table I. CLINICAL SIGNS* (*Continued*)

Brain Death	*Persistent Vegetative State*
"Survival"	
In terms of continued cardiac functioning	In terms of continued vegetative existence
Limited—hours to days	May be prolonged, days to years
Prolonged "survival" rare (4–6 weeks)	
Prognosis in Terms of Extent and Reversibility of Brain Damage	
Because of sequence of events described above (with permanent loss of brain blood flow) an accurate determination can be made, with an extremely high degree of certainty, within hours to days.	Accurate determination can be made within three to six months, often only after repeated examinations over a prolonged period of time.

* Reproduced with permission of Ronald Cranford, M.D.

COUNSEL. It is ethically permissible (perhaps obligatory) to discontinue all medical intervention when a patient shows the clinical signs of irreversible cessation of total brain function. This patient is dead, and medical interventions, even those which support breathing, are meaningless; none of the goals of medical intervention can be accomplished.

NOTE. Some Jewish Orthodox rabbis object to this position [cf. Bibliography 3.3]. Also, a few other ethicists express caution, even when agreeing in principle. The question of discontinuing life support for persons who do not meet this criterion but are in persistent vegetative state raises quite different ethical issues. These are discussed in Chapter 3.

NOTE. Discontinuation of life-prolonging therapy, decisions not to initiate certain treatments (such as cardiopulmonary resuscitation), and the determination of how much analgesia is necessary to relieve pain all require the use of *clinical discretion*. Indeed, the preliminary decision by the physician that the patient is irreversibly ill and dying also requires such discretion.

1.7.3 **Legal Issues.** Declaration of death, although usually done by a physician in accord with medical criteria, is a legal matter. Anglo-American common law sanctioned the criteria suggested by common sense and employed by doctors: the cessation of respiration and heartbeat. Many states have statutes that incorporate these criteria, and they are still commonly used by judges. In general, a physician who declares a person dead by employing the cardiopulmonary criteria, applied with due care, would be acting in accord with the law. In recent years, many states have passed "brain death statutes" (Table II). While these are stated in different ways, they agree in allowing the declaration of death to be based on another criterion, namely, the irreversible cessation of brain function. These statutes do not dictate the methods whereby this cessation is determined; they should be the most reliable clinical methods available at the time [cf. Guidelines, Bibliography 1.7]. A physician who applies these criteria with due care in a state that has a brain death statute acts according to the law. (Of course, cardiopulmonary criteria may and usually will be used in most cases; their use is not abrogated by brain death statutes.) In states without brain death legislation, a physician may apply brain death criteria as widely accepted good clinical practice, but with greater uncertainty about the legal implications. Where the statute exists, presumption favors the physician in difficult legal cases about the time and cause of death, e.g., when an inheritance is at issue, when an organ is removed for transplant, when criminal charges are pending against a person who attacked the decedent. The President's Commission for the Study of Ethical Problems in Medicine has recommended the adoption of a uniform statute for all states [1.7].

COMMENT. There are no unambiguous rules which dictate decisions in these matters. Decisions depend on clinical discretion. Perhaps the enthusiasm for brain death statutes among both philosophers and physicians reflects their desire for a rule to predetermine decisions with which they would otherwise be uncomfortable and insecure. But insecurity and discomfort and even terror are entirely appropriate emotions when one is confronted by the awesome and irreversible decisions concerning the life and death of another.

Table II. MODELS ADOPTED BY 25 STATES FOR STATUTORY DEFINITION OF DEATH

Kansas Model: Alternative Means for Determining Death[a]	*Capron-Kass Model: Brain Death Pronouncements Can Be Made Only When Heart and Lung Function Are Artificially Maintained*	*American Bar Association Model: Irreversible Cessation of Total Brain Function Equals Death*	*Uniform Brain Death Model Similar to ABA Model but Emphasizes Irreversible Cessation of Brain Stem Function*
Kansas 1970	Alaska 1974	California[b,g] 1974	Nevada 1979
Maryland 1972	Michigan 1975	Georgia[b,h] 1975	Wyoming[f] 1979
New Mexico 1973	West Virginia[c] 1975	Oklahoma 1975	
Virginia[b] 1973	Louisiana[g] 1976	Illinois[c] 1975	
Oregon 1975	Iowa[b] 1976	Tennessee 1976	
North Carolina[e] 1977	Hawaii[b,g] 1978	Idaho[b] 1977	
	Texas 1979	Montana 1977	
	Alabama[g] 1979	Arkansas[d] 1979	
		Connecticut[b,g,f] 1979	

[a] Essentially similar to AMA model bill.
[b] Use of brain-related criteria to pronounce death requires opinion of two physicians. In some instances (Virginia and Hawaii), one of these must be a specialist in neurology or neurosurgery.
[c] Brain-related criteria to be used only for purposes of the Anatomical Gift Act, i.e., for purposes of organ donation. In essence this places the law in the "Alternative Means" category.
[d] Also requires absence of spontaneous breathing.
[e] As amended in 1979; like Capron-Kass in some regards.
[f] Total brain function is defined as purposeful activities of the brain as distinguished from random activity.
[g] Physician who makes the determination of death may not participate in removal or transplantation of organs from the deceased.
[h] Permits but does not require death pronouncement with irreversible cessation of brain function.

Therefore, physicians will not find their problems of terminating therapy solved by legislative enactments (such as the California Natural Death Act or brain death statutes), by judicial pronouncements (Quinlan, Saikewicz, Fox), or by hospital ethics committees, although these may reflect the concerns of the community. Rather, a firm understanding of the goals of medicine, its appropriate ends, and the application of clinical discretion permit the physician to make reasonable, if not always perfect, choices in caring for patients. Imperfections and uncertainty are one of medicine's—and man's—eternal burdens.

1.7.4 **Termination of Therapy.** Any decision to terminate treatment or not to resuscitate should be accompanied by efforts to make the patient as comfortable as possible. The decision is to terminate *therapy,* that is, active interventions intended to cure or retard the course of a disease. It is not a decision to terminate *care,* i.e., medical, social, and psychological intervention to alleviate pain and to enhance the quality of the patient's last days. The medical proverb is pertinent: Cure sometimes, relieve occasionally, comfort always.

1.8 MEDICAL ETHICS COMMITTEES

Medical ethics committees have been established in recent years. They are useful for consultation regarding complicated cases. Legal, medical, and ethical ramifications of a decision can be explored. Different views regarding prognosis and indications for treatment can be exposed. Arguments about "quality of life" can be closely scrutinized (cf. Chapters 3 and 4). In particular, conflicts among family members or among the medical and nursing team can be mediated. Committee review may provide assurance that full and impartial consideration has been given to a difficult ethical decision. Committees should be used for consultation and review; they should not be substituted for the responsible decision of the attending physician.

1.9 THE THIRD MODEL: COPE (Chronic, Outpatient, Palliative, Efficacious)

CLINICAL EXAMPLE OF COPE MODEL. A 42-year-old woman with a strong family history of diabetes mellitus was first noted to have diabetes seventeen years ago when she presented with an episode of ketoacidosis during her first pregnancy. The pregnancy ended with a miscarriage. In the early years following her diagnosis, her diabetes was difficult to control. Although she complied with her dietary and medical regimen, she experienced frequent episodes of ketoacidosis and hypoglycemia, which necessitated repeated hospitalizations and emergency room care.

For the next ten years, however, her diabetes was well controlled, and she required hospitalization only twice: once for ketoacidosis associated with acute pyelonephritis and once when she was admitted electively in her eighth month of pregnancy and delivered a healthy baby.

She has been actively involved in her diabetic program. She is scrupulous about her eating habits and maintains an ideal body weight. She also is knowledgeable about the use of insulin and currently takes 40 units of NPH and 5 units of regular insulin each morning. On this program, her urine fractionals are negative, her fasting blood sugars are less than 120 mg per cent, and her two-hour postprandial sugars are usually below 160 mg per cent. She rarely experiences episodes of hypoglycemia. Seventeen years after the onset of diabetes, she appears to have no functional impairment from her disease. However, fundoscopic examination reveals a moderate number of microaneurysms, and urinalysis shows persistent proteinuria (less than 1 gram per day). She has no neurological symptoms or abnormal physical findings.

1.9.1 **The Clinical Features of the COPE Model.** We use the term COPE to describe ambulatory doctor-patient interactions in physicians' offices or outpatient clinics. The COPE model is the basic model for ambulatory care. In internal medicine and family practice, the ambulatory setting is where most patient–physician encounters occur. Many of these encounters are visits for checkups or for minor, self-limited illness. However, in the practice of internal medicine and to a lesser degree in family practice, many such visits are for the care and support of patients with chronic diseases. Indeed, the majority of internists' practice is concerned with chronic diseases such as hypertension and its sequelae, heart disease and strokes; arteriosclerotic cardiovascular disease and its complications; diabetes mellitus; osteoarthritis or rheumatoid arthritis; chronic abdominal problems such as irritable bowel syndrome or peptic ulcer disease; chronic bronchitis and obstructive pulmonary disease; and cancer. Even many of the acute problems that are brought to the internist's attention are superimposed on underlying chronic diseases. These conditions represent examples of the COPE model (*C*hronic, *O*utpatient, *P*alliative, *E*fficacious).

(a) *Chronic*. Each of these is a chronic condition in which the patient has lived with the disease, its symptoms, and its functional impairment, often for a long time. The patient is usually knowledgeable about the disease. Frequently, in the natural course of these chronic diseases, acute medical complications may develop that are related to the underlying disease.

> EXAMPLES. Acute pulmonary edema in chronic cardiac disease or gastrointestinal hemorrhage in portal hypertension related to cirrhosis of the liver are examples of acute complications of chronic diseases.

(b) *Outpatient*. In contrast to ACURE and CARE situations, most COPE conditions are managed in outpatient settings rather than in the hospital. This difference has important ethical implications. In the hospital, the physician and other hospital personnel have enormous power (both physical and psychological) to influence patient choices. However, in the outpatient setting, the patient is considerably more independent and powerful in interaction with physicians. In the outpatient setting, the patient's ultimate power may be wielded by simply severing contact with this particular physician or with all physicians.

(c) *Palliative*. For most of the chronic conditions being considered in the COPE model, definitive cure does not exist, and the physician can only palliate or soften the effect of the disease. Thus, symptoms and complications may be reduced (e.g., as in diabetes) but the underlying disease is not usually modified.

(d) *Efficacious*. Although cure is not a possibility in most COPE diseases, therapy is often effective in reducing symptoms (e.g., in rheumatoid arthritis), maintaining function (as in the diabetes example in 1.9) preserving patient dignity, and even in prolonging life (e.g., by treating chronic hypertension or chronic congestive heart failure).

1.9.2 **Medical Goals in the COPE Model.** In COPE medical situations, some of the goals of medicine are more important than others. Although preservation of life, preservation of function, and reduction in pain and suffering remain major goals, the goals of medicine may be restated in the COPE situation as follows:

(a) to use the arts of medicine, both by active intervention and, when necessary, by self-restraint, to assist the patient to live as independently and comfortably as possible.

(b) to use the art and science of medicine to minimize the patient's need for current and future medical intervention. This is done by emphasizing preventive medicine, health education and good health habits, personal responsibilities for health, and compliance with health regimens including, but not restricted to, medications.

1.9.3 **The COPE Model and Some Clinical Ethical Problems.** Although the outpatient setting in which COPE model situations occur is much less dramatic than the hospital setting in which ACURE and CARE models predominate, the possibility of clinical ethical problems exists. Unfortunately, because these situations lack the drama of life-and-death matters, physicians and patients may fail to recognize them as ethical problems. Ethicists rarely discuss them.

The COPE model is defined by the achievement of a doctor–patient accommodation in which the patient chooses to seek help from a particular physician and in which the physician agrees to care for the patient. There is a unique opportunity to achieve a doctor–patient accommodation through a process of negotiation in chronic, noncritical situations such as those in the COPE model. In ACURE or CARE situations, where the patient is often critically ill, negotiation and accommodation might be curtailed in order to attend to the patient's urgent medical needs. Also, the patient is clearly less capable of participating in negotiation.

The patient has greater control over COPE encounters than

ACURE or CARE encounters. The patient can define a problem as one needing a doctor's help, can initiate contact with a physician (or choose not to), and at any time can change physicians or drop out of the medical system entirely.

However, the physician is also party to achieving a doctor–patient accommodation. The physician's decision to enter such an arrangement is based on (a) ability to help the patient while (b) remaining loyal to norms of behavior associated with acting responsibly as a good physician.

In the COPE model there is a high level of personal interaction between physician and patient; relatively frequent encounters in the office or clinic, exchange of information about the patient's progress, and discussion of matters that go beyond the illness, such as family difficulties, money problems, and so forth. In this setting, expression of preferences by the patient and by the physician play a large part. Any ethical problems encountered in the COPE model are likely to revolve around differences and divergencies in preferences. The next chapter explores problems of this sort, particularly:

(a) The noncompliant patient [2.8]
(b) The problem patient [2.8.1]

BIBLIOGRAPHY

Annas, G. J. Beyond the Good Samaritan: Should Doctors Be Required to Provide Essential Services? *Hastings Center Report,* 1978, **8**(2):16.

Beauchamp, Childress, 1979: Chapters 4–5.*

Barber, B. Compassion in Medicine: Toward New Definitions and New Institutions. *N Engl J Med,* 1976, **295:**939.

Mack, E. Bad Samaritanism and the Causation of Harm. *Phil Pub Affairs,* 1980, **9:**230.

Kleinig, J. Good Samaritanism. *Phil Pub Affairs, 1976,* **5:**382.

1.1.2 *Clinical Discretion*

Adelman, H., Adelman A. Explorations Toward a Logic of Empirical

* Complete citations for abbreviated references appear at the end of the book under "General References."

Discovery: A Case Study in Clinical Medicine. *J Med Phil,* 1977, **2**:54.

Carlton, W. *"In Our Professional Opinion . . .": The Primacy of Clinical Judgment over Moral Choice.* Notre Dame, Ind.: University of Notre Dame Press, 1978.

Cassell, E. J. Preliminary Explorations of Thinking in Medicine. *Ethics in Science and Medicine,* 1975, **2**:1.

Churchill, L. R. Tacit Components of Medical Ethics: Making Decisions in the Clinic. *J Med Ethics,* 1977, **3**:129.

Engelhardt, H. T., Spicker, S. F., Towers, B. (eds.). *Clinical Judgment: A Critical Appraisal.* Boston and Dordrecht: D. Reidel, 1977.

Feinstein, A. R. *Clinical Judgment.* Baltimore: Williams & Wilkins, 1967.

Murphy, E. A. *The Logic of Medicine.* Baltimore: The Johns Hopkins Press, 1976.

Siegler, M., Goldblatt, A. D. Clinical Intuition: A Procedure for Balancing the Rights of Patients and the Responsibilities of Physicians. In *The Law-Medicine Relation: A Philosophical Exploration.* S. F. Spicker, J. M. Healey, H. T., Engelhardt (eds.). Boston and Dordrecht: D. Reidel, 1981.

1.1.3 *Goals of Medical Intervention*

Cassell, E. J. The Function of Medicine. *Hastings Center Report,* 1977, **7**(6):16.

Jonsen, A. R. Do No Harm. *Ann Intern Med,* 1978, **88**:827.

Kass, L. R. Ethical Dilemmas in the Care of the Ill. Part I, *JAMA* **244**:1811, 1980; Part II, *JAMA*, **244**:1946, 1980.

Kass, L. R. Regarding the End of Medicine and the Pursuit of Health. *The Public Interest,* Summer 1975, p. 11.

1.2.2 *The Uncertainties of Medicine*

Bosk, C. L. Occupational Rituals in Patient Management. *N Engl J Med,* 1980, **303**:71.

Fox, R. The Evolution of Medical Uncertainty. *Milbank Memorial Fund Quarterly/Health and Society,* 1980 **58**:1.

Gorovitz, S., MacIntyre, A. Toward a Theory of Medical Fallibility. *Hastings Center Report,* 1975, **5**(6):13; *J Med Phil,* 1976, **1**:51.

McNeil, B. J., et al. Primer on Certain Elements of Medical Decision Making. *N Engl J Med,* 1975, **293**:211.

Murphy, E. A. *Probability in Medicine.* Baltimore: The Johns Hopkins Press, 1979.

Pickering, G. Therapeutics: Art or Science? *JAMA,* 1979, **242**:649.

1.4 *CARE Model*

Tumulty, P. A. *The Effective Clinician.* Philadelphia: W. B. Saunders, 1973, Section C-4, "Patient with Incurable, Progressive and Fatal Disease."

1.5 *Decisions to Terminate or Withhold Intervention as Medically Inefficacious*

Amundsen, D. W. The Physician's Obligation to Prolong Life: A Medical Duty Without Classical Roots. *Hastings Center Report,* 1973, **8**(4):24.

Baier, K. The Ethics of Passive Euthanasia. *Crit Care Med* 1976, **4**:317.

Beauchamp, T. L., Davidson, A. The Definition of Euthanasia. *J Med Phil,* 1979, **4**:294.

Beecher, H. K. Ethical Problems Created by the Hopelessly Ill Patient. *N Engl J Med,* 1968, **278**:1425.

Cassem, N. H. Confronting the Decision to Let Death Come. *Crit Care Med,* 1974, **2**:113.

Cohn, H. Natural Death—Humane, Just and Jewish. *Sh'ma,* 1977, **7**(132):97.

Clouser, K. D. Allowing or Causing: Another Look. *Ann Intern Med,* 1977, **87**:622.

Clouser, K. D. "The Sanctity of Life": An Analysis of a Concept. *Ann Intern Med,* 1973, **78**:119.

Collins, V. U. Limits of Medical Responsibility in Prolonging Life: Guides to Decision. *JAMA,* 1968, **206**:389.

Connery, J. R. Prolonging Life: The Duty and Its Limits. *Linacre Q.,* 1980, **47**:151.

Foot, P. Euthanasia. *Phil Pub Affairs,* 1977, **6**:84.

Imbus, S. R., Zawacki, B. E. Autonomy for Burned Patients When Survival Is Unprecedented. *N Engl J Med,* 1977, **297**:308.

Lo, B., Jonsen, A. R. Clinical Decisions to Limit Treatment. *Ann Intern Med,* 1980, **93**:764.

Nelson, L. Primum Esse Utile. *Yale J Biol Med,* 1978, **51**:655.

Swazey, J. P. To Treat or Not to Treat: The Search for Principled Decisions. In Abernethy, 1980: 139.

Swiss Academy of Medical Sciences. Guidelines Concerning Assistance to the Dying. *Schweizrischen Akademie der Medizinischen Wissenshaften,* 1978, **108**:1169. *Hastings Center Report,* 1977, **7**(3):30.

Tagge, G. F., et al. Relationship of Therapy to Prognosis in Critically Ill Patients. *Crit Care Med,* 1974, **2**:61.

Temkin, O., Frankena, W. K., Kadish, S. H. *Respect for Life in Medicine, Philosophy and the Law.* Baltimore: Johns Hopkins Press, 1975.

Tendler, M. D. Torah Ethics Prohibit Natural Death. *Sh'ma.* 1977, **7**(132):97.
Veatch, R., 1976: Chapter 3.

1.5.1 *"Passive Euthanasia"*

For References, Cf. 3.3.

1.5.2 *Legal Liability*

Fletcher, G. P. Prolonging Life. *Washington Law Rev,* 1967, **42**:999. (In Gorovitz, 1976: 261; in Shannon, 1976: 189.)
Meyers, D. W. Legal Aspects of Medical Euthanasia. *Bioscience,* 1973, **23**:467.

1.6 *Orders Not to Resuscitate (No-Code Orders)*

Baron, C. H. The Dinnerstein Decision and 'No Code' Orders. *N Engl J Med,* 1979, **300**:264.
Liacos, P. Dilemmas of Dying. *Medicolegal News,* Summer 1979, **7**(3):4.
New York Academy of Medicine Statement on Measures Employed to Prolong Life in Terminal Illness. *Bull NY Acad Med,* 1973, **49**:349.
Optimum Care for Hopelessly Ill Patients: A Report of the Critical Care Committee of Massachusetts General Hospital. *N Engl J Med,* 1976, **295**:362.
Rabkin, M. T., et al. Orders Not to Resuscitate. *N Engl J Med,* 1976, **295**:364.
Robertson, J. Legal Criteria for Orders Not to Resuscitate: A Response to Justice Liacos. *Medicolegal News,* February 1980.
Schram, R. B., Kane, J. C., Roble, D. T. 'No Code' Orders: Clarifications in the Aftermath of Saikewicz. *N Engl J Med,* 1978, **299**:875.
Spencer, S. Code or No Code: A Non Legal Opinion. *N Engl J Med,* 1979, **300**:138.

1.7 *Brain Death*

Bernat, J. L., Culver, C. M., and Gert, B., On the Definition and Criterion of Brain Death. *Ann Intern Med,* 1981, **94**:389.
Black, P. McL. Brain Death I. *N Engl J Med,* 1978, **299**:338; Brain Death II. *N Engl J Med,* 1978, **299**:394.
Byrne, P. A., O'Reilly, S., Quay, P. M. Brain Death: An Opposing Viewpoint. *JAMA,* 1979, **242**:1985.
Cranford, R. E., Smith, H. L. Some Critical Distinctions Between Brain Death and the Persistent Vegetative State. *Ethics Sci Med,* 1979, **6**:199.

1.7 *Brain Death*

Defining Death: A Report on the Medical, Legal and Ethical Issues in Definition of Death. President's Commission on Ethical Problems in Medicine and in Biomedical and Behavioral Research. Washington D.C.: Government Printing Office, 1981.

A Definition of Irreversible Coma: Report of the Ad Hoc Committee of the Harvard Medical School to Examine the Definition of Brain Death. *N Engl J Med*, 1968, **205**:337.

Guidelines for the Determination of Death: Report of the Medical Consultants on Diagnosis of Death to the President's Commission on Ethical Problems in Medicine and in Biomedical and Behavioral Research. *JAMA*, 1981, **246**:2184.

Green, M. B., Wikler, D. Brain Death and Personal Identity. *Phil Pub Affairs*, 1980, **9**:105.

Jonas, H. Against the Stream. In Philosophical Essays. Englewood Cliffs, N.J.: Prentice-Hall, 1974.

Korein, J. (ed.). Brain Death: Interrelated Medical and Social Issues. *Ann NY Acad Sci*, 1978, p. 315.

Plum, F., Posner, J. B. *The Diagnosis of Stupor and Coma*. Philadelphia: Davis, 1980.

Refinements in Criteria for Determination of Death: An Appraisal. *JAMA*, 1972, **221**:48.

Ramsey, P. 1970: Ch. 2.

Stickel, D. L. The Brain Death Criterion of Human Death. *Ethics Sci Med*, 1979, **6**:177.

Veatch, R. M. 1976: Ch. 1–2.

Vieth, F. J., et al. Brain Death I: A Status Report of Medical and Ethical Considerations. *JAMA*, 1977, **238**:1851; Brain Death II: A Status Report of Legal Considerations. *JAMA*, 1977, **238**:1744.

Walker, A. E. An Appraisal of the Criteria of Cerebral Death. *JAMA*, 1977, **237**:982.

1.7.3 *Legal Issues*

Capron, A. M., Kass, L. A Statutory Definition of the Standards for Determining Human Death. *U Penn Law Rev*, 1972, **121**:87. (In Shannon, 1976: 137.)

Horan, D. J. Euthanasia and Brain Death: Ethical and Legal Considerations. *Linacre Q.*, 1978, **45**:248.

1.8 *Medical Ethics Committees*

May, W. Composition and Function of Ethics Committees. *J Med Ethics*, 1975, **1**:23.

Shannon, T. A. What Guidance from the Guidelines? *Hastings Center Report*, 1977, **7**(3):28.

Veatch, R. M. Hospital Ethics Committees: Is There a Role? *Hastings Center Report*, 1977, **7**(3):22.

2

PREFERENCES OF PATIENTS

2.0 This chapter discusses the preferences expressed by persons who seek or are in need of medical care. These preferences are often an important, and frequently a decisive, consideration in the ethical problems that arise in the course of care. The various issues and problems associated with the expression or the absence of preferences are discussed in the following order (a) the ethical, legal, and psychological nature of patient preferences; (b) competence and capacity to consent or refuse; (c) informed consent and refusal of treatment; (d) the "living will"; (e) proxy consent and "presumed consent;" (f) preferences of minors; (g) the noncompliant and "difficult" patient.

The ethical principle underlying the discussions of this chapter is the principle of autonomy. This ethical principle, widely endorsed in our culture, was forcefully expressed by John Stuart Mill:

> The only part of conduct of any one for which he is amenable to society, is that which concerns others. In the part which merely concerns himself his independence is, of right, absolute. Over himself,

his own body and mind, the individual is sovereign. (*On Liberty* [1859]. New York: Appleton-Century-Crofts, 1947, p. 10.)

The principle of autonomy has a legal counterpart in the right of self-determination. In American law, the legal right to self-determination has particular import for medical care. In 1914 Justice Cardozo wrote:

Every human being of adult years and of sound mind has a right to determine what shall be done with his body. [Schloendorff v. Society of New York Hospital.]

The most significant ethical and legal problem raised by the principles of autonomy and self-determination is the problem of "paternalism." Paternalism is defined as "the interference with a person's liberty of action justified by reasons referring exclusively to the welfare, good, happiness, needs, interests or values of the person being coerced" (Dworkin, 1972). Law can be paternalistic: the Food and Drug Act, which prohibits importation, prescription or manufacture of laetrile, has been passed with the intention of protecting the welfare of cancer patients. Medical practice has traditionally been strongly paternalistic: Physicians have often concealed diagnoses from patients "for their own good." The ethical question is whether paternalism is ever justified and, if it is, under what circumstances. This question is discussed in the sections on truthful disclosure [2.4] and refusal of treatment [2.5].

2.1 ETHICAL, LEGAL, AND PSYCHOLOGICAL SIGNIFICANCE OF PATIENT PREFERENCES

When there are medical indications for treatment, a physician normally proposes a treatment plan, which a competent patient may either accept or refuse. *An informed, competent patient's preference to undergo or to refuse medically indicated treatment is of great ethical, legal and psychological importance.* (EB: PATIENTS' RIGHTS MOVEMENT.)

2.1.1 **General Considerations.** Patient preferences are the legal and moral nucleus of a patient–physician relationship: In most circumstances the patient–physician relationship can be neither initiated nor sustained unless the patient desires it. Although the patient may need the assistance of a physician, it is important for physicians to remember that the patient, not the physician, has the primary legal and moral authority to establish patient–physician relationships. Patients, not physicians, are legally permitted to terminate the relationship at will; physicians who do terminate a relationship with a patient still needing help are held to certain moral and legal standards of behavior, e.g., giving timely warning and even helping the patient find another physician. In general, a competent adult has a right not to seek or permit any medical care, even if the medical intervention might be necessary to save his/her life. If a competent patient wishes to withdraw from and terminate a relationship with a physician, the patient has a legal and a moral right to do so. Furthermore, at various phases of medical decision-making, patient preferences are essential for competent clinical care. A physician who ignores, neglects, or disregards patient preferences when they are relevant may be violating legal, ethical, and professional expectations. (EB: THERAPEUTIC RELATIONSHIP.)

2.1.2 **Ethical Significance.** Patient preferences are ethically significant because they make explicit the values of self-determination and personal autonomy that are deeply rooted in the ethics of our culture. Autonomy is the moral right to choose and follow one's own plan of life and action. Respect for autonomy is the moral attitude that inclines one to refrain from interference with another's beliefs and actions. The recognition of patient preferences enhances the value of personal autonomy in medical care. In practice, however, many forces obstruct and limit the expression of patient preferences; such forces—the compromised competence of the patient, the informed consent process, the psychodynamics of the physician–patient interaction, the stress of illness—contribute to problems of clinical ethics considered in this chapter.

2.1.3 **Physicians' Respect for Patient Preferences.** This is essential to the development of a mature therapeutic alliance. Although patients have the legal and moral authority over physician–patient relationships, physicians have enormous power in these relationships. They can shape the course and the moral dimensions of medical care by their psychological dominance, specialized knowledge, and technical skills. The physician's power can, if misused, undermine the therapeutic relationship and destroy the fragile moral autonomy of the patient. This is not to deny that patients have important responsibilities in maintaining the relationship; still, illness and hospitalization preoccupy and even incapacitate some patients. Not all patients are equally affected by illness, but all are potentially vulnerable to a reduced level of functioning and of conscious interaction. Therefore, physicians must be particularly sensitive to the psychodynamics of patient preferences.

EXAMPLE. A 46-year-old woman with a family history of breast cancer visits her physician every six months for a breast examination. (Outwardly composed, she is in fact so frightened of breast cancer, from which her mother died, that she cannot bring herself to do self-examination.) On one visit the doctor notes a 2-cm mass in the left breast, and he recommends a biopsy. She refuses and abruptly terminates the visit. The physician notes in the record, "I recommended a biopsy and patient refused for unknown reason." He pursues the matter no further.

COMMENT. This physician, despite knowing the patient's history, obviously failed to comprehend the complex dynamics of this patient's reaction to the possibility of breast cancer. Since she had visited him frequently, there was ample opportunity to explore this matter.

2.1.4 **Legal Significance.** Patient preferences are legally significant because the Anglo-American legal system recognizes that each person has a fundamental right to control his own body and the right to be protected from unwanted intrusions or "unconsented touchings." An important judicial opinion states:

> Anglo-American law starts with the premise of thoroughgoing self-determination. It follows that each man is considered to be master of his own body, and he may, if he be of sound mind, prohibit the performance of life-saving surgery or other medical treatment. [Natenson v. Kline, 1960.]

The legal requirement of explicit consent prior to specific treatments protects the patient's legal right to control what is done to his own body. The documentation of the patient's consent also serves as a defense for the physician against a claim that the patient's rights had been violated.

In addition, patient preferences are significant because the law has considered the patient–physician relationship to be a sort of contract. Essential to a contract is the consent of both parties. The patient–physician "contract" is sometimes described in terms of a "fiduciary relationship" in which one party is held to a higher standard of performance than in an ordinary contract. The fiduciary, in this case the physician, has an obligation to protect the best interests of the person who has entrusted himself to his care. Despite this obligation, the patient's consent initiates the contract and sustains it by accepting the recommendations of the physician. The patient's withdrawal of consent can terminate it.

2.1.5 **Psychological Significance.** Patient preferences are psychologically significant because the ability to express preferences and have others respect them is crucial to a sense of personal worth. The patient, already threatened by disease, has a vital need for the sense of worth and control. Further, if patients' preferences are ignored or devalued, patients are likely to distrust and perhaps disregard physicians' recommendations. Patients' distrust of physicians endangers the therapeutic benefits that flow from a positive relationship. If patients are overtly or covertly uncooperative, the effectiveness of therapy is threatened. Furthermore, patient preferences are important because they may lead to the discovery of other factors—the patient's fears, fantasies, or unusual beliefs—that a physician should consider in prescribing or implementing treatment.

2.1.6 **Agreement of Preferences.** Physicians express their preferences to the patient by making recommendations regarding an appropriate course of care. Patients express their preferences to the physician by stating implicitly or explicitly their desire to be cared for, their acceptance of the physician's recommendations, and their hopes for satisfactory results. In most encounters between patients and physicians, these preferences will be in agreement: The physician will respond to the patient's preferences, and the patient will accept the physician's recommendations. In this way a therapeutic alliance which is ethically, medically, and emotionally satisfactory can be formed. However, there will be situations in which this agreement will be lacking, e.g., the physician may fail to elicit the preference of the patient or may fail to provide information about which the patient can express reasonable preferences. The patient may not express preferences, may not understand information provided, or may refuse, implicitly or explicitly, the recommendations. When discord appears, ethical problems are encountered. The following sections review the most common of these problems.

2.1.7 **Clinical and Moral Considerations of Treatment.** In most medical encounters, the medical indications for treatment and the patient's preferences will be in accord; the patient has presented himself/herself with the intention of being treated. This agreement does not eliminate other ethical dimensions of the treatment situation. The manner in which a consenting and cooperative patient is treated has moral aspects. An oncologist who informs her patient only about the technical aspects of chemotherapy fails to treat the patient as well as the disease. This failure is a clinical error on the part of the doctor who mistakenly believes that medical care can be reduced to mere technique, such as administration of drugs or performance of surgery. The moral error in such practices is a lack of respect for the patient as a person. Satisfactory communication can unify and deepen the moral integrity and technical achievements of the physician–patient relationship. The primary care practitioner is often responsible for ensuring that specialist colleagues and the patient communicate adequately with each other.

2.2 COMPETENCE AND CAPACITY TO CHOOSE

The preferences of a *competent,* informed patient to accept or refuse treatment should be respected. What is competence? The answer is very complex and often confusing. Physicians often misunderstand the notion of competency (usually by oversimplifying it or applying it to circumstances incorrectly). Competence is a commonsense concept that has acquired a technical, though somewhat imprecise, meaning in the law.

Competence in ordinary life may refer to mechanical or technical skills or intellectual or emotional capacities. It means a person is able to perform certain tasks and do so adequately or proficiently. In this sense it is heavily value laden, resting more on norms than on facts. The term "clinical competence," used to evaluate physicians, carries this meaning. In the law, competence usually refers to mental capacities, such as understanding, reasoning, and emotional stability, sufficient to appreciate the nature and consequences of such things as making a contract or a will, standing trial, or being a parent. *The terms "competence" and "incompetence" should be restricted to the legal status of a person: The person is judged, by proper legal authority, usually a judge, to be able or unable to understand the nature and consequences of decisions.* (Minors, of course, are not competent to conduct their own affairs, e.g., entering a contract, in terms of statutes that define the age of majority.) The degree of understanding required by the law will vary in relation to the task to be performed and the circumstances. It will be, in the last analysis, what satisfies the judge. If the person is judged "incompetent," a guardian or conservator is appointed to make decisions. The conservator may be limited to making only particular sorts of decisions, such as those concerning business affairs, for the ward. In other circumstances a conservator "of the person" is authorized to consent to medical treatment for the ward. In the legal sense then, a person may be declared incompetent in business or financial matters and yet remain legally competent to consent to or refuse medical care. Laws concerning competence, conservatorship, and guardianship vary from state to state. It should be clear that a judgment of competence or incompetence is the outcome of a specific legal process.

2.2.1 **Mental Capacity and Mental Incapacity.** In the medical care situation, competence may have yet another meaning. Persons in need of medical care sometimes appear disoriented, confused, obtunded, psychotic. The physician must determine whether they are capable of understanding their situation and making choices about it. *For such situations, we prefer the terms "mental capacity" and "incapacity," describing the functioning of sensory and mental powers to process data and to draw conclusions.* We use these somewhat novel terms in order to distinguish between the legal status of persons and the physician's assessment of behavior in the clinical setting. Incapacity, in this sense, can be developmental or pathological. Developmental incapacity refers to the immature mental processes of infants, children, and the developmentally disabled. Pathological incapacity arises from some permanent or temporary deficit in the psychophysiological processes, e.g., due to encephalopathy, senile dementia, or severe psychosis. A patient in coma or unconscious is clearly incapacitated; the person is apparently not perceiving self or world and apparently not understanding or reasoning about the situation. Beyond coma, unconsciousness, and such psychopathological states as catatonia, there is considerable disagreement about psychological criteria for capacity. Even if there were agreement about tests for capacity, the problems of application to particular cases would remain.

2.2.2 **Determination of Mental Capacity or Mental Incapacity.** The physician must determine whether or not the patient is incapacitated. This should be done by the standard clinical tests, either by the internist or by a consulting psychiatrist. A complete and orderly mental status examination should include:

(a) An evaluation of the patient's orientation to person, place, time, and situation
(b) A test of recent and remote memory and logical sequencing
(c) An assessment of intellectual capacity, that is, ability to comprehend abstract ideas and to make a reasoned judgment based on that ability
(d) An assessment of mood and affect, noting particularly suicidal ideation
(e) An examination of the content of thought and perception for delusions, illusions, and hallucinations
(f) An inspection of visible behavior, noting agitation or anxiety, as well as appetite, eating habits, and sleeping patterns
(g) A review of past history for evidence of a psychiatric disturbance that might affect the patient's current judgment

2.2.3 **Causes of Mental Incapacity.** Physicians may have good clinical reasons to suspect incapacity; appropriate tests may confirm incapacity. In the clinical setting the suspicion of incapacity is based on manifest phenomena, such as disorientation, confusion, and so forth. In addition to these behavioral evidences, the suspicion may be supported by the presence of a variety of physical conditions known to be associated with altered mental status. Table III lists conditions often causing delirium and dementia, the principal manifestations of altered mental status.

The suspected or confirmed presence of any of these conditions does not justify a judgment of incapacity in the absence of any behavioral manifestations. However, their presence does justify further investigation into the patient's capacity when unusual behavior is manifested. Also, unusual behavior should lead the physician to seek for the presence of these physical conditions. It is crucial to identify physical causes of altered mental states that can be reversed by medical treatment and to attempt to do so promptly.

2.2.4 **Psychological State.** The assessment of a patient's mental state may show adequate ability to process information and relatively normal emotional states. Still, a patient may exhibit certain psychological states which, while not pathological, may affect in subtle ways the ability to comprehend and choose. Anxiety and depression are often associated with illness. These can be increased almost to the point of pathology by the anticipation of surgery, unfamiliarity with hospital settings, absence of supportive family, and the like. Physicians must recognize that considerable distortion can be introduced into the relationship with patients by such reactions. It is imperative that the physician recognize these affective states and make efforts to compensate for them.

In our opinion these mental states do not constitute incapacity as such. They do indicate an impairment of good judgment. They require very special efforts at support and communication. The timing and manner of important decisions should be carefully adjusted to the patient's psychological condition so that these decisions can be made in the best possible emotional and psychological circumstances. In our opinion, physicians have a legal duty to respect the decisions of persons who are not incapacitated, even though they seem depressed or anxious. However, they have an ethical duty to do everything within

Table III. SOME CONDITIONS CAUSING DELIRIUM AND DEMENTING DISORDERS*

Category of Disease	*Delirium*	*Dementing Disorder*
Infectious	Meningitis Encephalitis Pneumonia	Chronic meningitis Tertiary syphilis Jakob-Creutzfeld disease
Intoxications	Abstinence drug states Delirium tremens Drug abuse	ETOH abuse Bromidism Chronic barbiturate intoxication
Metabolic	Hepatic encephalopathy Uremia Diabetic encephalopathy Endocrinopathies Porphyria Electrolyte abnormalities Dehydration	Hypothyroidism Cushing's disease
Neoplastic and vascular	Supratentorial lesions: brain tumor brain abscess subdural hematoma Subtentorial lesions: infarction tumor	Frontal lobe meningioma CVA
Traumatic	Concussions High CNS pressure	Chronic subdural hematoma Midbrain hemorrhage
Miscellaneous	Nutritional states Exogenous poisons Medications: steroids antihypertensives Postoperative states Sensory deprivation	Wernicke-Korsakoff disease Parkinsonism Huntington's chorea Multiple sclerosis Wilson's disease Normal pressure Hydrocephalus Pernicious anemia Folate deficiency

* With permission of Richard Crayne, M.D.

their power to counter the effects of depression and anxiety on the patient.

2.2.5 **Judgments Regarding Incapacity to Choose.** The following cases represent situations in which the question of the patient's incapacity might be raised.

CASE I. Mr. K. M., a 38-year-old, hard-driving business executive who had multiple cardiac risk factors (smoking, borderline hypertension, obesity), awakened from sleep with substernal chest pain and shortness of breath. His wife urged him to go to the emergency room or to call the physician, but he refused. Several nights later he awakened with even more severe chest pain. He had great difficulty catching his breath. At his wife's urging, he went to an emergency room, where an electrocardiogram demonstrated an acute, evolving anterior wall myocardial infarction. The patient was treated with low doses of morphine sulfate, and the pain resolved. As preparations were being made to admit the patient to the Coronary Care Unit, he informed the physician he did not wish to be admitted to the hospital and was going to return to his home. His wife attempted to dissuade him from this decision. He refused to listen to her advice. The physicians at the hospital explained to the patient the risks of his returning to his home rather than being monitored in the setting of a Coronary Care Unit and strongly urged admission. At this point, the patient showed no signs of mental illness or lack of comprehension. He had no life-threatening cardiac rhythm disturbances and, at the time of presentation at the emergency room, he was not in left-sided heart failure. He returned home. [Cf. 1.3–1.3.3.]

COMMENT. The patient's condition is dangerous, but without a basis for suspecting incapacitation the patient's refusal is decisive. The physician may consider it a regrettable decision but should respect it. Of course, the physician may pursue the problem, attempting to seek reasons for the refusal, to persuade, and to engage the help of others, such as the patient's wife. Education and vigorous persuasion constitute an ethical approach to refusal by a person capable of choice; coercion does not.

CASE II. In the case presented at 1.3, Mr. ACURE presents

with signs and symptoms suggestive of bacterial meningitis. He is informed of the diagnosis and told he will be admitted immediately to the hospital for treatment with antibiotics. He abruptly refuses hospitalization and treatment without giving any reason. The physician explains the extreme dangers of going untreated and the minimal risks of treatment. The young man persists in his refusal. Apart from this strange adamancy, he exhibits no evidence of mental derangement or altered mental status. [Cf. 1.3–1.3.3.]

COMMENT. There is no overt clinical evidence to support a judgment that ACURE is incapacitated. The physician might *presume* altered mental status due to fever or metabolic disturbance, but mere presumption, in the absence of behavior, is inadequate to justify a conclusion that Mr. ACURE is incapacitated. Nevertheless, the refusal of a treatment so necessary and entailing minimal risk, especially without offering a reason, is enigmatic. The physician has a moral obligation to pursue the matter further. It is important, at this point, to state strongly that a refusal of treatment should not, in and of itself, be considered the act of an incapacitated person. Physicians will sometimes say any refusal of lifesaving treatment is "crazy" and assume the person to be incapacitated. We believe that in addition to the refusal there should be clinical evidence or solid medical reason to justify the judgment of incapacity. The ethical problem in this case may not be whether the patient is incapacitated but whether the serious medical need of a person whose capacity to choose appears intact should be treated contrary to that persons's wishes. The case, therefore, is further discussed and some conclusions drawn under Refusal of Treatment [2.5].

CASE III. T. D., a 73-year-old man, has gangrene in his left toes. Several physicians confirm the diagnosis and recommend amputation. The gangrene is not an imminent threat to his life, but the infection is slowly spreading from his toes through his foot. If an amputation is not performed, it is expected that septicemia will occur and an amputation might, at a later stage of illness, be insufficient to prevent the patient's death. [Cf. 1.4–1.4.4.]

T. D. is oriented to time and place and his long-term memory is reliable. He has a sense of humor and engages in a coherent and reasonable conversation—except about his gangrenous foot. He knows his foot is sore and swollen, but he insists that it is getting better. Pain medication, after several weeks of severe pain without medication, may account for his belief that his foot is getting better. He is admitted to the hospital as an involuntary psychiatric patient after falling asleep while smoking and setting his couch on fire. While in the hospital, he vacillates about whether to permit an amputation. At first he consents to, and then refuses, the recommended surgery. After he is discharged, his foot gets worse. When examined by physicians, psychiatrists, and lawyers, T. D. denies he has gangrene and denies anyone told him that he had gangrene (even though he had repeatedly been told). When asked what he would do if he did believe he had gangrene, he immediately says he would tell the doctor to amputate. A judge concludes T. D. is incompetent to refuse the needed amputation.

COMMENT. In this case, T. D. did not accept—because of mental deficiency, psychological denial, or delusional belief—that he did in fact have gangrene and needed an amputation. Some of the important considerations that lead to a conclusion to operate contrary to the patient's expressed preferences are:

(a) T. D.'s statement that he *would* consent to amputation if he believed he really had gangrene
(b) T. D.'s obvious vacillation between accepting and rejecting surgery
(c) The nature of the life-threatening illness, as opposed to some less serious disease
(d) The relatively short time available in which to make a decision

COUNSEL. In our opinion, the life-threatening aspects of the illness and the likelihood that death could be prevented with amputation, *along with the patient's statement that he would accept surgery if he really had gangrene,* would together constitute decisive ethical grounds to allow surgeons to proceed to amputate. This ethical conclusion leads them to seek proper legal authority.

NOTE. A crucial element in the decision was Mr. T. D.'s statement that he would accept amputation if he did have gangrene. This statement is picked out from all of Mr. T. D.'s other statements as representative of his "true" wishes—what he would wish if he did not have delusional beliefs. The physicians have seized upon this statement because it conforms to the reality they see and supports the decisions they believe reasonable. In fact, the statement itself might flow from the complex psychological process that produces the denial. This picking and choosing among a patient's statements to find the "right" one, or the assumption that certain statements mean something the physicians wish to hear, is problematic. On the one hand, it represents an honest attempt to acknowledge the patient's preferences; on the other, it comes close to a rationalization for the doctors' getting their own way. In this case, we believe the decision to be ethically correct and the assumption of Mr. T. D.'s true wishes not unreasonable. The ethical correctness, it must be noted, rests not only on this assumption but on all four factors mentioned under "Comment" taken together. However, we must note that picking and choosing can be, in some cases, an unvarnished act of medical paternalism.

CASE IV. Mrs. L. O. is a 73-year-old woman who has lived alone for the last 12 years. She is known by neighbors and by her doctor to be fiercely independent and determined. She has no signs of senile dementia nor, apart from some eccentricities, does she show any abnormal behavior. Her medical problem is the same as that presented in Case III. She adamantly refuses amputation, although she insists she is aware of the consequences and accepts them. [Cf. 1.4.–1.4.4.]

COMMENT. Mrs. L. O. cannot be considered incapacitated to make choices in her own behalf; there is no evidence to support such a judgment. On the contrary, the evidence confirms she enjoys considerable capacity. She has no delusional belief and exhibits no vacillation.

COUNSEL. After being assured that she does understand her condition and its prognosis, her physician should put aside the thought of seeking a judicial determination of incompetence. Treatment of Mrs. L. O. should be limited to appropriate medical management. Continuing efforts to persuade her to accept amputation might be made.

2.2.6 **Evaluating Capacity to Choose in Relation to the Need for Intervention.** Usually a patient's capacity is not seriously questioned unless the patient decides to refuse or discontinue treatment. In such situations tests of capacity to consent might be applied. These tests can range from the simplest tests of mental status available to any physician to the more sophisticated evaluations applied by a psychiatrist or clinical psychologist [2.2.2]. It has been suggested that the stringency of the test should vary with the seriousness of the disease and urgency for treatment; the degree or level of capacity required for decision-making varies with the extent and probability of risk, with the extent and probability of benefit, *and* with consent or refusal. Thus, for example, a patient might need only a low level of capacity to *consent* to a procedure with substantial, highly probable benefits and minimal, low probability risk, but a high level of capacity to *refuse* the same treatment. If Mr. ACURE were confused and disoriented, his consent to treatment can be accepted; his refusal should arouse suspicions (as it did) of incapacity (Roth *et al.,* 1977).

2.2.7 **Waxing and Waning Capacity.** Certain pathological conditions, such as organic brain syndrome, are characterized by a movement in and out of mental clarity. A patient may be assessed as incapacitated at one time but later appear clear and oriented.

EXAMPLE. Patient CARE, with multiple sclerosis, is now hospitalized. In the morning he is able to converse for short periods with doctors, nurses, and his wife; in the afternoon he confabulates and is disoriented to place and time. In both conditions he expresses various preferences about his care, which are sometimes contradictory. In particular, when questioned about surgical placement of a tube to prevent aspiration, he says no in the morning and, in the afternoon, speaks confusedly and repeatedly about having the tube placed.

COUNSEL. This waxing and waning is itself the manifestation of pathology. The patient should be considered to have impaired capacity. The expression of preferences in such a state should not be considered *determinative,* unless there is consistency in the preferences expressed during periods of clarity.

2.2.8 **Unusual Beliefs.** Patients will sometimes express beliefs that appear to others as unusual and, on occasion, allow these unusual beliefs to guide their choices of medical care. Unusual beliefs are of many sorts: unsupportable claims about the physical world (e.g., the flat-earth believers), claims about health and medical treatment that are unverified (e.g., benefits of macrobiotic diet), theological beliefs of a sectarian nature that represent a minority interpretation of a broad religious tradition, as do the Jehovah's Witnesses or Christian Scientists, or that are idiosyncratic, such as a person or group maintaining God disapproves of drug therapy. Persons encountering others who hold unusual beliefs are often tempted to call them "crazy" and their beliefs "irrational." Without debating the meaning of irrational or arguing the psychiatric significance of unusual beliefs, we wish to note that the mere fact of adherence to an unusual belief is not in and of itself evidence of incapacity. In the absence of clinical signs of incapacity, such persons should be considered capable of choice. On occasion, however, their choices will have significant effect on their health and medical care. (For refusal of care on the grounds of unusual beliefs, e.g., the Jehovah's Witnesses belief about blood transfusion, cf. 2.5.1.)

2.2.9 **Medical-Legal Decisions for Incapacitated Persons.** When a physician does have good grounds for considering a person incapacitated, what can be done legally to authorize medical treatment? There are several courses of action open to the physician. (1) If the medical treatment is not necessary to save the patient's life, the physician can honor the person's wishes and refrain from treatment in the immediate situation. Psychiatric or other forms of help might be sought. Many courts have upheld the refusal of treatment by persons who were mentally incapacitated. (2) If treatment is necessary to save the patient's life, the physician might proceed to treat on the basis of the legal doctrine of implied consent [2.7.1]. (3) The physician might detain and treat the patient involuntarily under authorization by a particular statute in the jurisdiction. These statutes are usually quite specific, allowing the physician to treat against the patient's will only when the patient is suffering mental disease and when the patient is a danger to self or others [2.7.2]. (4) The physician or some other party, such as the hospital administrator, can seek authorization to treat a legally incompetent patient from the appropriate court in the jurisdiction.

2.3 INFORMED CONSENT

In recent years emphasis has been placed upon informed consent as a central element in the ethical and legal relationship between patient and physician. When making a diagnosis and recommending treatment, the physician is expected to provide sufficient information about the patient's condition and the recommended treatment—its benefits, risks, and alternatives—to enable the patient to make a responsible decision to accept or reject the recommendations. While the law has long maintained that absence of consent to medical treatment could warrant a charge of criminal battery, only in recent years has the legal doctrine of *informed* consent been elaborated by the courts. Failure to obtain informed consent has led to civil litigation for damages rather than criminal prosecutions for battery. Defects in consent have been construed as negligence, which constitutes one kind of malpractice.

2.3.1 **Disclosure of Information to Patient.** The practice of informed consent is significant because it reinforces the value of personal autonomy. The right of persons to choose how they will live and the extent to which others will enter into that life in various ways depends on their information about themselves, their understanding of that information and their free and willing acceptance of the role of others in their life.

In addition, the exchange of information establishes the interpersonal relationship between physician and patient on which our conception of the rights and duties of each party rests. The patient provides certain information to the physician; the physician analyzes that information and, in turn, informs the patient about his/her condition. This creates reciprocity between patient and physician. A reciprocal relationship between autonomous persons is the ideal of the ethical relationship between physician and patient. However, this ideal is often not attained. When it is not, ethical problems will often appear.

2.3.2 **Failure to Disclose Information to Patient.** The informed consent doctrine requires the physician to provide sufficient information for a patient to be able to make a rational and responsible decision. Just as the information the patient provides the physician is essential to enable the physician to make an accurate diagnosis, so also the physician's disclosures to the patient are necessary to enable the patient to express an intelligent preference. If the physician fails to disclose alternative forms of treatment, the patient is precluded from expressing a preference among them. If the physician fails to disclose the risks and side effects of a proposed treatment and the risk of refusing treatment, the patient lacks information that might influence a decision whether or not to undergo treatment. Thus, for a physician to fail to disclose information relevant to a patient's decision undermines the patient's legal and moral rights and the reciprocity of their relationship. Furthermore, subsequent discovery of this failure may threaten patient trust in the physician or contribute to problems of patient compliance with prescribed treatment procedures. The disclosure requirements for informed consent, therefore, have not only legal and moral but also clinical implications. Proper and sufficiently complete disclosures reinforce the relationship of reciprocity. (EB: INFORMED CONSENT IN THE THERAPEUTIC RELATIONSHIP.)

Patients may derive benefits other than making choices from information about their condition. Using educational materials may not only inform patients but also increase confidence in their physician, enhance patient satisfaction and compliance, and may even improve outcome. It is tempting in the face of the rigors of clinical practice and the vulnerability and confusion of patients to short-cut informed consent. Appropriately timed and modulated disclosures can strengthen the physician–patient relationship by increasing trust and respect and by reassuring the patient of the physician's personal concern. Abrupt and cryptic answers to legitimate concerns or even irrational fears of patients may be more threatening to some patients than realistic, even if painful, truth. For others, uncertainty is more tolerable than detailed information. Informed consent requirements may be modified by the patient who consciously chooses to limit the information received. The more common situation, however, is a patient who wants to know more but is afraid to ask. When the truth is or should be told, it is important that physicians do not tell more than they know, e.g., by making premature disclosures, or tell it in a manner that inflicts unnecessary distress. Tact, timing, and style are as important as accuracy in truth-telling.

2.3.3 **Comprehension.** The phrase "informed consent" stresses the giving of information. Most legal discussions of informed consent emphasize the amount and kind of information the doctor provides. Consent forms list risks and benefits (sometimes in excessive detail). However, the comprehension of the patient is fully as important as the providing of information, and it poses several ethical problems. Is it the physician's duty to assure comprehension? If so, how can comprehension be assured? How does the physician deal with persons of limited intelligence, of different cultural and linguistic backgrounds? Is it possible to communicate medical information comprehensibly?

Some studies and many anecdotes suggest that the comprehension by patients of medical information is not outstanding. At the same time studies and impressions suggest that methods of communication are poor and that little effort is made to overcome barriers to comprehension.

The physician has an ethical obligation, based on the reciprocal nature of the patient–physician relationship and upon the autonomy of the patient, to make reasonable efforts to assure comprehension. Explanations should be given clearly and simply; questions should be asked to assess understanding. Written instructions or printed materials should be provided. Educational programs for patients with chronic disease (COPE and CARE) should be arranged.

2.3.4 **Informed Consent: Definition and Standard.** Informed consent is defined as the willing and uncoerced acceptance of a medical intervention by a patient after adequate disclosure by the physician of the nature of the intervention, its risks and benefits, as well as of alternatives with their risks and benefits. Disclosure is judged "adequate" by two standards: (a) information that is commonly provided by competent practitioners in the community or the specialty; (b) information that would allow reasonable persons to make prudent choices in their own behalf. The former standard (a) allows more room for physician discretion; it is also more susceptible of being distorted by excessive paternalism. The latter standard (b) leans more on the autonomy of the patient. The latter standard has become the one favored in court decisions of recent years. A responsible practitioner would do well to use the latter (b) as the standard for disclosure.

2.3.5 **Stringency.** The moral and legal obligation of disclosure also varies in terms of the situation; it becomes more stringent and demanding as the treatment situation moves from emergency through elective to experimental. In some emergency situations, very little information can be provided. Any attempt to inform may be at the price of precious time. Ethically and legally, information can be curtailed in emergencies. When treatment is elective, much more information should be provided. Finally, detailed and thorough information should accompany any invitation to participate in research, particularly if the research maneuver is not directed to the patient's therapy [cf. 4.6].

2.3.6 **"The Therapeutic Privilege."** Difficult ethical decisions arise not only about how detailed information should be but also whether to withhold information which the physician judges might be harmful to the patient or which the patient is likely to misinterpret. The major legal decisions that have strongly stressed the duty of informed consent based upon patient autonomy have also acknowledged the so-called "therapeutic privilege." This terminology is somewhat misleading. It is not so much that physicians enjoy a special prerogative to withhold the truth. Rather, in a legal proceeding they may offer a defense to the charge of failing to inform by stating they did so "in the patient's interest."

> A disclosure need not be made beyond that required within the medical community when a doctor can prove by a preponderance of the evidence he relied upon facts which would demonstrate to a reasonable man the disclosure would have so seriously upset the patient that the patient would not have been able to dispassionately weigh the risks of refusing to undergo the recommended treatment. [Cobbs v. Grant, 1972.]

Another important legal decision states a caveat: The privilege does not accept the paternalistic notion that the physician may remain silent simply because divulgence might prompt the patient to forgo therapy the physician feels the patient really needs (Canterbury v. Spence, 1972). The justification for withholding information is discussed under "Truthful Disclosure" [2.4].

2.3.7 **Difficulties about Informed Consent.** Many physicians feel the informed consent requirement imposes upon them an undesirable and perhaps impossible task. It is considered undesirable because adequately informing a patient takes too long and might create unnecessary anxiety. It is considered impossible because no medically uneducated and clinically inexperienced patient can truly grasp the significance of the information the physician must disclose. Even physicians, when they are patients, may not comprehend information germane to their own illness. Selective hearing because of denial, fear, or preoccupation with illness may account for failure to take in what one might otherwise understand. For these reasons physicians sometimes dismiss the informed consent requirement as a meaningless but bureaucratically necessary ritual. However, it should be kept in mind that the physician is legally required only to make appropriate disclosures and to attempt to communicate, not to achieve the impossible. It is not legally required that physicians disclose *all* risks, e.g., those of taking aspirin or of drawing blood. The physician must strive to communicate as much as is reasonably possible in a given situation. Relatively little is known about how much patients do understand, how much information they wish, or whether information is detrimental, although most studies show that patients do desire information and that little or no harm is known to have resulted from disclosure.

2.4 TRUTHFUL DISCLOSURE

Communications between physicians and patients should be truthful, that is, statements should be in accord with facts. If the facts are uncertain, that uncertainty should be acknowledged. Deception, by stating what is untrue or by omitting what is true, should be avoided. These ethical principles govern all human communication. However, in the communication between patients and physicians, certain ethical problems arise about truthfulness. Does the patient really want to know the truth? What if the truth, once known, causes harm? Might not deception help by providing hope? In the past, answers to these questions by physicians have been ambiguous. Thomas Percival's *Medical Ethics* (1802) states, "To a patient . . . who makes enquiries, which, if faithfully answered, might prove fatal to him, it would be a gross and unfeeling wrong to reveal the truth. His right to it is suspended . . . because, its beneficial nature being reversed, it would be deeply injurious to him, to his family and to the public." Laypersons, on the other hand, have often expressed a different opinion. Samuel Johnson berates doctors, "You have no business with consequences. You are to tell the truth . . . of all lying I have the greatest abhorrence of this because I believe it has been frequently practiced on myself." (EB: TRUTH TELLING.)

CASE I. A 65-year-old man comes to his physician with complaints of abdominal pain which is persistent but not extreme. Studies show metastatic cancer of the pancreas. The patient has just retired from a very busy career and has made plans for a round-the-world tour with his wife. Should his diagnosis be revealed to him?

COMMENT. In recent years, commentators on this problem have moved away from the more ambiguous position of traditional medical ethics toward a strong assertion of the right of the patient to the truth. Their arguments are:

(a) There is a strong moral duty to tell the truth that is not easily overridden by speculation about possible harms.

(b) The patient has a need for the truth if he or she is to make rational decisions about actions and plans for life.

(c) Concealment of the truth is likely to undermine the patient–physician relationship. In cases of serious illness, it is particularly important that this relationship be strong.

(d) Tolerance of concealment by the profession may undermine the trust that the public should have in the profession. Widespread belief that physicians are not truthful would create an atmosphere in which persons who fear being deceived would not seek needed care.

(e) Suspicion on the part of the physician that truthful disclosure would be harmful to the patient may be founded on little or no evidence. It may arise more from the physician's own uneasiness at being a "bearer of bad news" than from the patient's inability to accept the information.

(f) Recent studies have shown that the majority of patients with diagnoses of serious illness wish to know the diagnosis. This counters the presumption that patients do not want to know. Similarly, recent studies are unable to document harmful effects of full disclosure.

COUNSEL. (a) The considerations in favor of truthful disclosure are, in our opinion, conclusive in establishing a strong ethical obligation on the physician to tell the truth to patients about their diagnosis and about the condition and its treatment.

(b) Speaking truthfully means relating the facts of the situation. This does not preclude a manner of relating the facts that is measured to perceptions of the hearer's emotional resilience and intellectual comprehension. The truth may be "brutal," but the telling of it should not be. Measured and sensitive disclosure is demanded by the ethical principle of respect for the automomy of the patient. It reinforces the patient's ability to deliberate and choose; it does not overwhelm this ability.

(c) If some facts have no implications for the patient's deliberation and choices, they need not be revealed. *Example:* Liver function studies revealed that the patient with cancer of the pancreas had elevated alkaline phosphatase with normal bilirubin. Even though this suggests the development of jaundice in the future, the physician judged this information irrelevant to the patient at this time.

CASE II. Mr. S. P., a 55-year-old teacher, has had chest pains and several fainting spells during the last three months. He reluctantly visits a physician at his wife's urging. He is very nervous and anxious and says to the physician at the beginning of the interview that he abhors doctors and hospitals. On physical examination, he has classic signs of tight aortic stenosis. The physician wishes to recommend cardiac catheterization. However, given his impression of this patient, he is worried lest full disclosure of the risks of catheterization would lead the patient to refuse the procedure.

COMMENT. In this case, the anticipated harm is much more specific and dangerous than the harm contemplated in the previous case. Hesitation about revealing a grim prognosis arises from fear the news may cause distress and even depression. Hesitation about revealing the risks of a diagnostic or therapeutic procedure is based on the fear the patient will make a judgment detrimental to health and life. Also, in this case, there is better reason to suspect this patient will react badly to the information than the patient in Case I.

COUNSEL. The arguments in favor of truthful disclosure apply equally to this case and to the previous one. Whether or not catheterization is accepted, the patient will need further medical care. This patient needs, above all, the benefits of a good and trusting relationship with a competent physician. Honesty is more likely to create that relationship than deception. Also, the physician's fears about the patient's refusal may be exaggerated. In addition, studies indicate that very few patients do refuse recommended procedures and that almost all patients desire disclosure. Finally, the physician might be concerned about the family's reaction if Mr. S. P. died unexpectedly during catheterization.

2.4.1 **Completeness of Disclosure.** Disclosure of options for treatment of a patient's condition should be complete, including the options which the physician recommends and also other options which the physician may believe are less desirable but which are still medically reasonable. In so doing, the physician should make it clear why these other options are less desirable. However, it might be asked whether the obligation of truthful disclosure requires telling a patient even of those interventions that are not medically reasonable, but which a patient may wish to consider.

CASE I. A 41-year-old woman has a breast biopsy which reveals cancer. The physician's best treatment of this premenopausal woman would be a mastectomy, axillary node dissection, and perhaps adjuvant chemotherapy. Should he also describe simpler procedures which he judges less suitable for this woman, such as a lumpectomy or mastectomy without axillary node dissection?

COUNSEL. The entire range of options should be explained with a careful delineation of the risks and benefits of each. There is no ethical prohibition against making a strong, persuasive argument in favor of the option the physician considers best. Persuasion, however, should leave the patient free to choose, even if the physician believes she may choose the less effective option.

CASE II. The same as Case I. Should the physician also reveal the existence of "unorthodox therapies," such as laetrile?

COUNSEL. The physician is trained in the medical management of illness. The obligation to disclose extends to all those forms of management that a competent practitioner might consider reasonable in terms of the current standards of the art and science of medicine. There is no obligation to disclose the existence of interventions of any other sort. It is, however, permissible to reveal the existence of unorthodox therapies. It may be advisable to do so if the physician believes the patient may be tempted to seek these treatments. In such a case it is imperative the physician explain the risks of unorthodox treatments and strongly advise against them. (EB: ORTHODOXY IN MEDICINE.)

2.4.2 **Placebos.** Concealing the nature of an intervention may sometimes be thought to contribute to its efficacy. This is so with "placebo" remedies. Is the use of placebos contrary to the obligation to truthful disclosure?

Placebo is defined as "any therapeutic procedure which is objectively without specific activity for the condition being treated" (Shapiro, 1954). This must be distinguished from the placebo effect, "the psychological, physiological, or psychophysiological effect of any medication or procedure given with therapeutic intent, which is independent of or minimally related to the pharmacologic effects of the medication or to the specific effects of the procedure and which operates through a psychological mechanism" (Shapiro, 1959). The placebo effect is known to take place as the result of many different influences: faith in the physician, administration of a medicine that the physician believes to be effective pharmacologically but is not, or actions of the physician that are not in themselves therapeutic, such as taking a history or performing a diagnostic test. Thus, the placebo effect may take place without deliberate deception; a placebo may not be a "false" or "fake" medicine. In the broader sense, in which no deception is involved, the placebo and the placebo effect are significant features of medical practice.

The problem of deception arises when the physician knows that the intervention does not have the objective properties necessary for efficacy and when the patient is kept ignorant of this fact. *Examples:* "yellow" pills for premenstrual tension or weekly shots of vitamin B_{12} for fatigue casually diagnosed as "tired blood." In some such cases, the deception is an outright moral offense, being motivated solely by the desire to keep the patient's fees or to "get the patient off my back." In other cases placebo deception may raise a genuine ethical question. The duty not to deceive seems to conflict with the duty to benefit without doing harm.

CASE I. A 73-year-old widow lives with her son. He brings her to a physician because she has become extremely lethargic and often confused. The physician determines that, after being widowed two years before, she had difficulty sleeping and had been prescribed hypnotics and that she now is addicted. The physician determines the best course would be to withdraw her from her present medication by a trial on placebos.

CASE II. A 62-year-old man has had a total proctocolectomy and ileostomy for colonic cancer. There is no evidence of remaining tumor; the wound is healing well and the ileostomy is functioning. On the eighth day after surgery, he complains of crampy abdominal pain and requests medication. The physician first prescribes antispasmodic drugs, but the patient's complaints persist. The patient requests morphine which had relieved his postoperative pain. The physician is reluctant to prescribe opiates. She believes the pain is psychological and knows that opiates will cause constipation. She contemplates a trial of placebo.

COMMENT. Any situation in which placebo use involves deliberate deception should be viewed as ethically perilous. The strong moral obligations of truthfulness and honesty prohibit deception; the danger to the patient–physician relationship (which is the most important nondeceptive placebo) advises against it. In those situations, however, when deceptive placebo use seems indicated, its ethical use rests on the following conditions: (1) The condition to be treated should be known as one that has high response rates to placebo, e.g., mild mental depression or postoperative pain; (2) the alternative to placebo is either continued illness or the use of a drug with known toxicity, e.g., monoamine oxidase inhibitors or morphine; (3) the patient wishes to be treated and cured, if possible; (4) the patient insists on a prescription.

COUNSEL. (1) When the above conditions are present, it is ethical to use a "deceptive" placebo. This is justified because, in an important sense, the placebo is known to be an effective agent, is harmless (although there can be placebo toxicity), and is an alternative to a more harmful drug. (2) The physician may justifiably state that this medicine (the placebo) is being given as a trial and that it is as likely to clear up the problem as any other drug. (3) If the desired effect does not appear within a reasonable time, the placebo should be discontinued. (4) It is imperative that any physician who uses a placebo be acquainted with the literature on the mechanism of the placebo effect, on the personality of placebo reactors, and on alternatives to placebo use. (5) The physician must not forget that the strong bond of trust between patient and physician is the most powerful placebo and that deception, if discovered, can destroy that bond. Short-term goals should not be traded for the long-term goal of continuing care for the health of the patient.

Thus, we consider the use of a placebo in Case I is not justified. The patient is not demanding. The problem of addiction should be confronted directly. There will be ample opportunity to develop a good relationship with this patient. Subsequent discovery of deception might undermine this relationship. Use of placebo in Case II is ethically permissible. The patient is demanding relief. Morphine is dangerous. A short trial of placebo may be effective in relieving pain and avoiding harm. Also, the cause of this late postoperative pain may be masked by use of opiates.

2.5 REFUSAL OF TREATMENT BY PERSONS WITH CAPACITY TO CHOOSE

Persons who are apparently informed and are not incapacitated sometimes refuse recommended treatment. When the treatment is elective, ethical problems are unlikely. However, if care is judged necessary to save life or manage serious disease, physicians may be confronted with an ethical problem: Does the physician's responsibility to help the patient ever override the patient's freedom? This problem is sometimes called the problem of paternalism, which is defined as overriding the preferences of a person in order to benefit that person or to prevent him/her from being harmed. (EB: RIGHT TO REFUSE MEDICAL TREATMENT.)

CASE. In the ACURE case [1.3] a young man presented with signs and symptoms suggestive of bacterial meningitis. When he was told his diagnosis and told he would be admitted to the hospital for treatment with antibiotics, he refused, without giving a reason. The physician explained the extreme dangers he was running in going untreated and the minimal risks of treatment. The young man persisted in his refusal. Other than this strange adamancy, he exhibited no evidence of mental derangement or altered mental status.

COMMENT. In this case the initial consent for diagnosis was implicit in the young man's presenting himself at the clinic. However, the patient's enigmatic refusal introduced an incongruence between medical indications and patient preference. It might be argued that the physician should simply permit the patient to refuse treatment since the patient showed no objective signs of incompetence. However, in the ACURE model in which the risk of treatment is low and the benefit is high and the risk of nontreatment is high and the "benefits" of nontreatment are low, it is ethically obligatory for the physician to probe further to determine why the patient desires to refuse treatment. Despite the explanation given, has the patient somehow failed to understand and appreciate the nature of his condition or the benefits and risks of treatment and nontreatment? If the patient understands the explanation, is he denying that he is ill? Or is he acting on the basis of some unexpressed fear, mistaken belief, or irrational desire? Through further discussion with the patient some of these questions might be answered. Assume, however, there is no evidence that the patient fails to understand and nothing emerges to indicate denial, fear, mistake, or irrational belief. Some might then ask, should the patient's enigmatic refusal be respected? Or, since his medical condition is so serious, should treatment proceed even against the patient's will? This case poses a genuine ethical conflict between the patient's personal autonomy and the paternalistic values which favor medical intervention. A clinical decision must be made quickly to treat or release the patient; good ethical reasons can be given for either alternative.

COUNSEL. This patient's refusal is truly enigmatic. There is no evidence of incapacity to choose due to altered mental state (although the patient's high fever might lead the physician to suspect some derangement). Further, there is no expression of an "unusual belief," e.g., a religious objection to antibiotics. The patient simply refuses and will provide no reason for his refusal. Given both this enigmatic refusal and the urgent, serious need for treatment, we counsel the patient be treated, even against his will, if this is possible. Should there be time, legal authorization should be sought. In offering this counsel, we have come down, with some reluctance, in favor of paternalistic intervention at the expense of personal autonomy. Our reluctance stems from the unwillingness to violate the liberty of another. It is overcome by the consideration that something essential is missing in this case. It is difficult to believe this young man wishes to die. The conscientious physician faces two evils: to honor a refusal which might not represent the patient's true preferences, thus leading to the patient's death, or to override the refusal in the hope that, subsequently, the patient will recognize the benefit. This is a genuine moral dilemma: The principle of beneficence and the principle of autonomy seem to dictate contradictory courses of action. In medical care, dilemmas cannot merely be contemplated; they must be resolved. Thus, we resolve it in favor of treatment against the wishes of this patient.

FURTHER COMMENT. In this case, we accept as ethically permissible the unauthorized treatment of an apparently competent person. In Case I [2.2.5], we allowed Mr. K. M., a man with a myocardial infarction, to leave the hospital. We would consider attempts to restrain him ethically impermissible. What considerations lead us to these apparently inconsistent conclusions?

(a) The medical indications are significantly different. Mr. ACURE has a critical disease, and low-risk treatment will be effective in preventing serious harm. There is an opportunity for complete achievement of all medical goals. The patient with the MI resembles ACURE cases in many respects: The patient suffers from an acute, critical problem. However, unlike Mr. ACURE's problem, this critical episode is not directly treatable nor reversible. Observation is advisable in order to be able to intervene in case of life-threatening arrhythmias or heart failure. However, observation, requiring admission, may itself be risky since it may increase the anxiety of an already anxious man resisting hospitalization.

(b) The consent situation is significantly different. In neither case is there behavioral evidence of incapacity. In both, the common psychological mechanism of denial impairs good judgment. However, in the case of Mr. K. M., the refusal takes place after a full disclosure of the problem and its risks. There has been opportunity to discuss, persuade and argue. He responds that he feels better and wants to go home. He has business that cannot be delayed. In Mr. ACURE's case, discussion is peculiarly truncated. Efforts to discuss are met with flat refusal. Yet he has willingly come to be treated. There is a strong suspicion that some crucial element of this negotiation is missing. It is that suspicion which leads the physicians, given the medical situation, to treat him against his wishes.

(c) In fact, something *was* missing. Mr. ACURE's mother had died several years ago of an anaphylactic reaction to penicillin. Mention of antibiotics had triggered a psychological response of denial, which manifested itself in a refusal without reason. (Indeed, the patient had no recall of these events when recovered.) The practical circumstances of his particular illness drew the physicians in the direction of rapid, perhaps slightly hasty, treatment. The physicians may have acted hastily and not very well, from a technical viewpoint. They did not have the time or the inclination to understand the patient's inarticulate refusal of penicillin. In this situation, if the physicians had been able to fathom the reason for the patient's refusal, i.e., an unarticulated fear of an anaphylactic reaction to pencillin, they might have been able to treat him with other and more appropriate antibiotics than they in fact used. In the case described, ampicillin was among the antibiotics employed and, fortunately, the patient did not experience the penicillin drug reaction.

(d) The case illustrates that physicians are often pressured by circumstances to make decisions before all relevant information is known. Thus, the rightness or wrongness of the clinical decision always must be assessed in terms of what the clinician knew or should have known at the time of the decision. In this case the physician *should* have known more. There is a tendency in medicine—in evaluating the rightness of both clinical and ethical decisions—to base such assessments on data that become available long after the decision had to be made. We include this complex and troubling case to illustrate how actual situations do, at times, yield ambiguous results. One can only strive to render decisions that are as fully and as carefully analyzed as the circumstances permit.

2.5.1 Refusal on Grounds of Unusual Belief

CASE. Mr. G. comes to a physician for treatment of peptic ulcer. He says he is a Jehovah's Witness. He is a firm believer and knows his disease is one that may eventually require administration of blood. He quotes the Biblical passage on which he bases his belief: "That ye abstain from meats offered to idols and from blood . . ." (Acts 15:28). The physician inquires of her Episcopal clergyman about the interpretation of this passage. He reports, after some research, that no

Christian denomination except the Jehovah's Witnesses takes it to prohibit transfusion. The physician considers Mr. G.'s belief both unreasonable in view of his health needs and unfounded in religious tradition. She also considers his preferences impose an inferior standard of care. What sort of "contract" should the physician make with this patient? (EB: BLOOD TRANSFUSION.) [Cf. 1.3–1.3.3.]

COMMENT. (a) As a general principle, the unusual beliefs and choices of other persons should be tolerated if they pose no threat to other parties. The ethical principle of autonomy requires that these beliefs and choices be respected, even though they appear mistaken to others. If, however, unusual beliefs do pose a threat to others it is ethically permissible and even obligatory to prevent harm by means commensurate with the imminence of the threat and the seriousness of the harm. Courts have, in recent years, upheld the legal right of Jehovah's Witnesses to refuse lifesaving transfusions. Courts have, however, intervened to order blood transfusions for the children of Jehovah's Witnesses. As Justice Holmes stated, "Parents may make martyrs of themselves, but they are not free to make martyrs of their children." Similarly, some courts have ordered transfusions even for adult Jehovah's Witnesses who were pregnant or whose death would leave children bereft of a mother or father.

(b) Refusal of blood transfusion differs in a significant way from a refusal of all therapy or of recommended treatments (e.g., the cases in 2.2.5 of the young man with meningitis and the man with myocardial infarction). The Jehovah's Witnesses acknowledge the reality of their illness and desire to be cured or cared for; they simply reject one modality of care. Physicians may feel this limitation involves them in substandard and incompetent medical care. This is the essence of the ethical problem posed by the Jehovah's Witness.

(c) The physician's inquiry about the interpretation of the Biblical passage is interesting. Presumably, she would feel more comfortable with a belief she knew to be part of her own religious tradition. Also, it might show an inclination to consider "conscientious beliefs" as those which are instilled in persons by God or religious authority (as the American courts long did with conscientious objectors to war). It is our opinion that the validity of a belief in terms of an orthodox tradition is not relevant. Rather, the sincerity of those who hold it and their ability to understand its consequences for their lives is the relevant issue in this sort of case.

COUNSEL. (a) Jehovah's Witnesses cannot be considered incapacitated to make choices unless there is clinical evidence of such incapacity. This evidence should be developed as rigorously as for any other case of suspected incapacity. Anecdotes suggest physicians may be inclined to sweep the Jehovah's Witnesses into the category of the incapacitated because of their unusual belief. On the contrary, these persons are usually quite clear about their belief and its consequences. It is a prominent part of their faith, insistently taught and discussed. Witnesses have a long history of standing by this belief. Thus, while others may consider it irrational, adherence is not, in itself, a sign of incapacity.

(b) If the Jehovah's Witness comes as a medical patient, the eventual possibility of the use of blood should be discussed and a clear agreement worked out between physician and patient about treatment in that eventuality. It should be learned whether the patient rejects autotransfusion and dialysis as well as blood and blood products. The availability of blood substitutes should be discussed; under no circumstances should the physician resort to deception. A physician who, in conscience, cannot accept being held to an inferior or dangerous standard of care should withdraw from the case.

(c) If the Jehovah's Witness is in need of emergency care and refuses blood transfusion, the refusal should be considered decisive unless there is some clinical evidence of incapacity to make a responsible decision. Should the patient, who is known to be a confirmed believer, be incapacitated, it can be presumed that the refusal represents the person's true wishes. If little is known about the patient and his status as a believer cannot be authenticated, treatment should be provided. In the face of uncertainty about personal preferences, it is our position that response to the patient's medical need should take ethical priority.

2.5.2 **Refusal of Information.** Persons have a right to information about themselves. Similarly, they have the right to refuse information or to ask the physician not to inform them. Some patients may prefer to trust the doctor to make the proper decisions. If this is clearly the patient's preference, it should be respected. On occasion, it will cause an ethical problem.

CASE. In the CARE case [1.4] the patient with multiple sclerosis had shown little interest during the early years of his illness in learning about the possible course of his disease. He even refused several offers by the physician to discuss this. However, on one of his repeated admissions for treatment of urinary tract infections, he states that, had he known what his life would be like, he would have refused permission for treatment of other life-threatening acute problems. The patient's mental status is difficult to evaluate; some think he shows signs of early dementia. Should he have been informed of his prognosis at an earlier time even though unwilling to engage in such discussions with his physician?

COMMENT. In this case we are concerned with what the physician communicates and should communicate about diagnosis and, particularly, prognosis. Should the physician override the patient's stated preference not to know about his condition? Should physicians withhold unpleasant information about prognosis to protect the patient from depression or other negative, potentially damaging emotions? Or should the patient be told, as soon as a reliable diagnosis has been made, enough to maximize his opportunity to plan his life in the face of future prospects? Although it is tempting to withhold information to protect the patient, perhaps a better alternative would be to give the patient general information sufficient to indicate the seriousness of his condition as well as the uncertainty about the time, the severity, and the extent of the problems that MS can cause. The middle ground avoids the extremes of withholding too much too long or disclosing too much too soon. Considerable discretion is required to find the proper balance of disclosure and tact. Furthermore, the disclosures made as the condition worsens must be adjusted in the light of the impairments to the patient's competence. In some cases of late-stage MS an associated dementia appears. Thus it would be advisable to make disclosures before the patient's capacity is so severely impaired that he cannot understand.

COUNSEL. Again we have a difficult case in which unpleasant but unavoidable moral choices must be made. Here we opt for more rather than less disclosure, especially because the condition, though untreatable, is long-lasting. Thus the patient's long-term moral autonomy is respected more by providing as much information as possible to enable him to make more choices while he is physically and mentally able to learn coping mechanisms in advance. The short-term gains of ignorance are outweighed by the long-term benefits of knowledge.

2.6 THE LIVING WILL

In recent years the document known as the living will has come into use. Its popularity has been fostered by a group called Concern for Dying. The term "living will" is somewhat misleading, since a "will," properly speaking, is effected after the death of the person who has made it. Also, the legal status of living wills is unclear. Nevertheless, many individuals prepare these documents in advance of the onset of serious illness as directions to their physicians concerning their medical treatment when they are dying. These documents typically contain such statements as "In case of serious illness from which I am unlikely to recover, I do not wish to be kept alive by heroic or extraordinary measures. I fear death less than the indignity of dependence and deterioration." The living will is a person's attempt to extend the expression of his/her preferences into a future when the actual expression will be impossible or difficult.

The living will represents evidence of the preferences of the patient. As in the case of any evidence, the meaning of a living will must be interpreted, its authenticity verified, and its application to the particular situation assessed. Living wills are not legally binding instruments. In some jurisdictions, legislation has been enacted to grant individuals some rights in this respect. California's Natural Death Act was enacted in 1976, followed by similar legislation in nine other states as of 1980.* Even where a document of this sort has some legal authority, the physician to whom it is directed must interpret it in the light of the patient's condition.

CASE I. A 70-year-old woman with severe hypertension suffers a stroke resulting in extensive paralysis. Her sister brings to the hospital a signed and witnessed living will, dated one year earlier. It contains the words, "I fear death less than the indignity of dependence and deterioration." The patient is currently unable to communicate. She is intubated and has cardiac arrhythmias. Should the physician, on becoming aware of her living will, extubate her? Should no-code orders be written in anticipation of cardiac arrest? [Cf. 1.4–1.4.4.]

CASE II. Mr. CARE, the patient with multiple sclerosis, is now hospitalized. He has suffered several respiratory arrests due to aspiration. His mental status is poor. He shows signs of organic brain syndrome. A question is raised about surgical placement of a tracheostomy tube. The patient's wife shows the physician a newspaper clipping describing the living will, with the note attached, "I am dictating to my wife my approval of this living will. I want it to apply to me when necessary." Is this sufficient to direct the physician not to take measures to prevent another respiratory arrest?

COMMENT. In both cases, evidence of personal preference is being offered. In the first case there can be no doubt about the authenticity of the document, although its interpretation in the situation is difficult. The eventual effects of the stroke cannot be clearly predicted at this time; the extent to which the patient will experience "the indignity of dependence and deterioration" is unknown. Thus respect for her wishes is best manifested by continuing indicated medical treatment until her prognosis can be determined more clearly. In the second case there may be some question about the authenticity of the evidence, although the application is much clearer. The patient suffers from a lethal disease and is now in its terminal stages. Prevention of death by

* Arkansas, Idaho, Kansas, Nevada, New Mexico, North Carolina, Oregon, Texas, Washington.

intermediate measures would only prolong an inevitable dying process. The expression of the patient's preferences, even though some doubt of its authenticity may exist, is helpful evidence for the clinician in considering whether to refrain from further intervention.

COUNSEL. (a) When presented with a living will by a patient, discuss its meaning and implications fully with the patient. Learn what the patient means by vague expressions such as "heroic and extraordinary measures" or "dependence and deterioration." In the first case the patient, who did recover with very little residual deficit, stated that she meant "she did not want to be a vegetable stuck with a lot of tubes."

(b) If discussion with the patient is not possible, make reasonable efforts to determine the authenticity of the document; e.g., ask relatives about the circumstances of its composition and about other expressions of preferences by the patient in conversations, letters, and the like. Examine the interests of other parties in the care of the patient [4.2.3]. Interpret the meaning of the stated preferences in light of the medical indications for treatment [1.1.3] and the prognosis for future quality of life [3.1–3.1.4].

(c) Be aware of the exact legal meaning of such documents in the state in which you are practicing.

2.6.1 **Extraordinary and Ordinary Measures.** The terms "extraordinary" and "ordinary" appear in documents such as the living will. They are also frequently used in discussions about withholding or withdrawing life-supporting medical interventions. Often, the term "extraordinary" is used interchangeably with such terms as "heroic" or "unusual" measures. These usages are confusing and usually not very helpful in determining what should be done. However, Roman Catholic medical ethics, where the "ordinary–extraordinary" distinction originated, attempts to give these terms a more precise meaning. In this system the terms "ordinary" and "extraordinary" *do not* refer to the state of medical art (e.g., in 1925 blood transfusion was "extraordinary"; in 1960 chronic hemodialysis was "extraordinary''; today both are ''ordinary''). Rather, the ''extraordinary'' nature of any treatment, regardless of how common and accepted as medical practice, refers to its impact on the personal, social, and even economic life of the patient and the patient's family. Roman Catholic moralists proposed that persons had a moral obligation to preserve their lives and care for their health, but that this moral obligation demanded only the use of ''ordinary'' means:

> Extraordinary means of preserving life are all medicines, treatments, and operations, which cannot be obtained or used without excessive expense, pain or other inconvenience for the patient or for others, or which, if used, would not offer a reasonable hope of benefit to the patient. [Kelly, G., Medico Moral Problems. St. Louis: The Catholic Hospital Association, 1958, p. 135.]

It was left to the patient, with the advice of doctors, to determine what treatments were ''extraordinary'' in this sense. The statement of Pope Pius XII remains the rule for Catholics and was recently reaffirmed:

> Normally one is held to use only ordinary means according to circumstances of persons, places, times and cultures, that is, means that do not involve pain or burden for oneself or another. [Pope Pius XII, 1958; The Prolongation of Life, 1958; Pope John Paul II, Declaration on Euthanasia, June 29, 1980.]

2.7 PROXY CONSENT

When a patient is thought to be incapacitated to refuse treatment—or even to consent to treatment—it is a common mistake to suppose a family member may consent on behalf of the patient. In most states the law *does not* permit family members —unless they have been legally authorized by court order granting guardianship to do so—to consent to or refuse medical care on behalf of an adult family member, incapacitated or not. In addition, mere suspicion of incapacity does not give physicians the authority to treat the patient against the patient's wishes unless a determination of incompetence has been legally obtained according to local laws and regulations, and an authorization to treat has been granted by court order or by the consent of the patient's guardian or conservator. [Cf. 1.3–1.3.3, 2.2, 4.2.]

2.7.1 **Implied Consent.** In some life-threatening emergency situations, patients are unable to express their preferences or to give their consent because they are unconscious or in shock. Physicians undertake lifesaving treatment without the express consent of the patient. It is often said this practice is legally justified by "implied consent": The patient can be presumed to want treatment and would give consent if able to do so. Still, implied consent is a legal fiction, inferred by the law from circumstances. It provides the physician with a defense against a subsequent charge of battery (although it may not defend against charges of negligence if the emergency treatment falls below acceptable standards of care). From the ethical point of view, the principle of beneficence, which prescribes that a person in serious need must be helped by one who can do so (without harm or great inconvenience to the helper), justifies initiating treatment in life-threatening emergencies.

2.7.2 **Statutory Authority to Treat.** In all jurisdictions, statutes exist which authorize the physician to hold a person for treatment against the will of that person. These statutes pertain to persons who suffer or are suspected of suffering from mental disease, and the treatment authorized is treatment for mental disease. In addition, the person must be considered a danger to self or others. The statutes do not apply to medical or surgical treatment as such (except provisions regarding involuntary treatment of communicable diseases in some states). However, in some situations both mental disease and medical problems may be present.

EXAMPLE. A 30-year-old man, known to the ER staff as psychotic and alcoholic, is brought to the hospital by a friend. He has been drinking and taking heroin and is hallucinating that Viet Cong are attacking him. He is breathless, has fainted twice in the last hour, and is incontinent of urine. He says his heart is breaking through his chest. Still, he says he has got to leave the hospital because it is being bombed. The admitting resident writes in the chart, "I noted hallucinations and psychotic ideation, thus, I am putting the patient on a medical hold and keeping him in the hospital for observation. Diagnosis: paroxysmal supraventricular tachycardia. Medications: haloperidol, digitalis. Further evaluation: assess electrolytes." [Cf. 1.3–1.3.3.]

COMMENT. The question is whether the statutory "medical hold" allows medical treatment as well as treatment for mental illness. Each state's statute and local interpretations must be consulted for an answer. In general, the statutes seem to refer to mental illness alone as the justification for involuntary commitment and to its treatment as the sole permitted intervention. The question is probably not legally important if the treatment is lifesaving. In that case the legal doctrine of implied consent would suffice. If not lifesaving, but urgent and highly advisable, the physician is placed in a somewhat unclear situation. A clinical assessment of incapacity is made, but the patient has the legal right to refuse care unless declared incompetent. The use of the "medical hold" for medical as well as psychiatric treatment may be technically illegal, but it appears to make ethical sense.

2.7.3 **Consent of Minors.** Persons who are younger than the statutory age of consent (age 18 in all states) may seek the care of a physician. If their medical problem is not an emergency, such persons can be treated only with the consent of their parents. However, there are several exceptions.

(a) Almost all jurisdictions now have special provisions for the treatment of certain conditions without the consent of the minor's parents. These conditions are usually drug abuse and venereal disease (contraception, abortion, and mental illness are sometimes included, sometimes specifically excluded). Physicians should be aware of the provisions of the law in the jurisdiction in which they practice.

(b) The emancipated minor is a young person who lives independently of parents, physically, financially or otherwise. Married minors, those in the armed forces or living away at college are considered emancipated. They may request treatment and be treated without parental consent.

(c) The legal concept of "mature minor" is being increasingly invoked. A mature minor is one who is below statutory age and who is still dependent upon parents but who appears able to make reasoned judgments. These young persons pose something of a quandary to the physician from whom they seek care. On the one hand, they appear able to decide for themselves; on the other, their parents remain legally responsible for them. Legal authorities conclude the physician may respond to their requests under the following conditions:

(i) The patient is at the age of discretion, by which is meant 15 or older, and appears able to understand the procedure and its risks sufficiently to be able to give a genuinely informed consent.

(ii) The medical measures are taken for the patient's own benefit (i.e., not as a transplant donor or research subject).

(iii) The measures can be justified as necessary by conservative medical opinion.

(iv) There is some good reason, including simple refusal by the minor to request it, why parental consent cannot be obtained.

COUNSEL. A physician may treat a minor without parental consent if the minor is emancipated or if there is statutory authorization for certain sorts of treatment. If the minor does not fit either category but is capable of understanding and consent, the physician may treat under the conditions mentioned above.

In the case of the mature minor, however, the physician should inquire, if possible, about the reasons for the young person's unwillingness to communicate with parents. Steps should be taken, if the minor is willing, to attempt reconciliation or to solve the problem in a mutually satisfactory manner. Confidentiality should be maintained.

Physicians who honor the requests of mature minors are at some theoretical legal peril. However, "no decision can be found within the past 20 years in which a parent recovered damages, even in the absence of a minor treatment statute, for treatment of a child over the age of 15 without parental consent" (Holder, 1977, p. 145).

A request for irreversible sterilization from a mature minor should probably never be honored. The legal reasons for this are the peril of suit by parents and by the minor at a later date. There are also statutory and regulatory prohibitions against sterilization of minors in certain federal programs and in many states. The ethical reason for refusal rests on the presumption that even a mature minor cannot comprehend the implications of this procedure as well as the likelihood of doing great harm.

2.8 FAILURE TO COMPLY WITH MEDICAL REGIMEN

The patient–physician relationship can be disrupted when patients who seek or need care fail to follow recommendations. This lack of accord between physician preferences and patient preferences is commonly called noncompliance.

> CASE. At 1.9 the COPE model was presented. This model represents a patient with chronic disease who is treated as an outpatient with therapies that are palliative and efficacious. The COPE case described a woman with diabetes mellitus diagnosed seventeen years ago. For the first seven years after the diagnosis she had frequent episodes of ketoacidosis and hypoglycemia, even though she followed her dietary and medical regimen. For the next ten years her diabetes was well controlled. Now consider the following developments in that case. After a stormy divorce, the patient has changed in several ways. In the three years following her divorce, she has gained 60 pounds and often has not taken her insulin medication. She also has been drinking alcohol excessively and is often drunk. During these years, she has required frequent admissions to the hospital for diabetic complications including: (a) ketoacidosis, (b) nonketotic hyperosmolar state, (c) traumatic and poorly healing foot ulcers, and (d) alcohol-related problems. While in the hospital, her diabetes is easier to manage, but even while in the hospital she is frequently found in the cafeteria eating excessively. On several occasions she has abused alcohol while in the hospital, and at those times blood alcohol levels in excess of 200 mg per cent were detected. Soon after discharge from the hospital, her diabetic control lapses.

Her physician is frustrated by her case. He blames the recurring medical problems on the patient's unwillingness to participate actively in her own care. The physician tells her she could easily control her diabetic problem by merely resuming health habits she had pursued three years previously, i.e., by losing weight, by taking her insulin regularly, and by drinking alcohol in moderation. The patient is not averse to changing her life style but on discharge from the hospital she continues her poor health habits. The physician urges her to have a psychiatric consultation. She agrees. The psychiatrist suggests a behavior modification program, which proves unsuccessful in changing her behavior. Finally, aversion therapy is suggested. Her physician hesitates to advise her to participate in this program.

She continues to require hospitalization lasting seven to ten days every month or two. After ten years of working closely with this patient, the physician considers withdrawing from the therapeutic relationship because he senses he is no longer able to help the patient. The patient resists this suggestion. She complains the physician is merely trying to punish her for her alcoholism.

COMMENT. Patients such as Mrs. COPE are very frustrating to those who attempt to care for them. Occasionally the physician will accuse the patient (in words or in attitude) of being irresponsible. The patient engages constantly and apparently willfully in behavior that poses serious risk to health and even to life. Such patients place great strain on the doctor–patient relationship; often the accommodation between doctor and patient founders because of the strain.

Mrs. COPE's doctor contemplated withdrawing from her case. He judged she was simply irresponsible and that her behavior undermined the care he was attempting to provide. "Why keep this up?" he said. "It's useless. Whatever I do, she undoes." Is persistent irresponsibility relevant to an ethical decision to withdraw from a case? Can it ever be decisive?

NOTE. The accusation of irresponsibility can be an example of the ethical fallacy of "blaming the victim"; the actual fault may lie with a more powerful party who finds a way to lay the blame for his own failure on the ones who suffer its effects. The poor, for example, were accused of lack of ambition by industrialists who paid paltry wages for wretched work. Similarly, the apparent irresponsibility of patients may be an impression created by the failure of a physician to educate, support, and convey personal concern and interest in the patient. It may be more than an impression: Persons may be rendered incapable of caring responsibly for themselves by the way their physician deals with them. An excessive paternalism may stifle responsibility, while a lack of personal concern may encourage noncompliance.

However, there may be cases in which the physician is not at fault; every effort has been made to educate, support, encourage. What then is the physician's responsibility?

COUNSEL. This patient's failure to comply with her medical regimen compromised her medical care. Noncompliance in asymptomatic diseases such as hypertension—in which the consequences of such behavior (e.g., stroke, myocardial infarction, or death) are statistical and far off—seem to be entirely a matter in which the patient is in control of the situation. The physician and society must use techniques of education to encourage the patient to desire treatment for hypertension. However, the situation presented in 2.8 is different in that many of the episodes of noncompliance result in avoidable medical problems which must be dealt with (sometimes as life-threatening emergencies) by the physician. The correct response is to deal with such problems exclusively in terms of the medical indications and not to make moral judgments about the merit or utility of treating an alcoholic, diabetic patient with expensive medical resources (such as intensive care units or skin grafts for foot ulcers.) [Cf. 3.2.4–3.2.6; 4.4.4–4.5.4.] Nevertheless, on rare occasions physicians may decide that no further treatment is indicated precisely because the patient's persistent behavior is so contrary to the goals of treatment [2.8.2].

It is important to decide whether the patient is acting voluntarily or involuntarily. Most noncompliant behavior is voluntary in the sense that the patient demonstrates no signs of pathological behavior. They either choose to ignore the regimen in favor of other behaviors they value more than health (a goal that might not seem very urgent or immediate) or fail in compliance because of such factors as irregular routine, complicated regimen, habitual forgetfulness, or poor explanation by the physician. Some noncompliance arises from profound emotional disturbance and ambivalence.

(a) If the physician judges that noncompliance arises from the patient's persistence in voluntary health risks, reasonable efforts at rational persuasion should be undertaken. If these fail, it is ethically permissible for the physician to adjust therapeutic goals and do the best in the circumstance; it is also ethically permissible to withdraw from the case, after advising the patient how to obtain care from other sources [2.9.1–2.10].

(b) If external circumstances are the source of noncompliance, help should be provided to improve these circumstances. Many helpful stratagems have been suggested to correct obstacles of this sort.

(c) If noncompliance arises from psychological pathology, the physician has a strong ethical obligation to remain with the patient, adjusting treatment plans to the undesirable situation. Professional assistance in treating the pathology should be sought. The physician will experience great frustration, but the frustration is not, in itself, sufficient to justify leaving the patient. Additional circumstances, however, may contribute to a justification. These are discussed below.

2.8.1 **The Problem Patient: Noncritical.** Noncompliance occurs in situations where the results, while harmful to the health of the patient, are not critical.

> CASE. Consider that the patient presented in 2.8 was admitted for in-patient treatment of her obesity with a protein-sparing modified fasting regimen. She was found repeatedly in the cafeteria cheating on her diet. Her physician made reasonable efforts to persuade her to change her behavior.

COUNSEL. It would be ethically permissible for the physician to abandon therapeutic goals and to discharge the patient from the hospital. These goals were unachievable because of the patient's failure to participate in the treatment program.

2.8.2 **The Problem Patient: Critically Ill.** Is it ever justifiable to discharge a "problem" patient who has a critical illness requiring in-hospital treatment? Just as we believe that noncritically ill patients can be discharged if they repeatedly frustrate physicians' efforts to provide needed medical assistance, we also believe that the noncooperation which directly counters the physician's effort can justify discharging a patient who is critically ill and in need of care. The situation, however, is more serious and requires added considerations before a decisive conclusion can be reached.

CASE. R. A., a chronic intravenous drug abuser, is admitted for the third time in three years with a diagnosis of infective endocarditis. Three years before, he required mitral valve replacement for pseudomonas endocarditis, and one year ago he required replacement of the prosthetic valve after he developed staph aureus endocarditis. He now presents again with staph aureus endocarditis of the prosthetic valve.

After one week of antibiotic therapy, he continues to have positive blood cultures. He consents to open heart surgery to replace again the infected mitral valve. For ten days postoperatively (four in the intensive care unit) he is cooperative and compliant with his management and antibiotic treatment. On this treatment he becomes afebrile, and blood cultures are negative.

He then begins to behave badly. He leaves his room and stays away for hours, often missing his dose of antibiotics. On several occasions a urine screening test demonstrates the presence of opiates and quinine, suggesting that he is using illicit narcotics even while being treated for infective endocarditis. On two separate occasions he punches nurses who scold him for being away from his room without permission. On the eleventh postoperative day he is discovered by hospital security guards in his bathroom selling injectable narcotics to another patient. His roommate in the hospital had observed these dealings for several days, but the patient had threatened to kill the roommate if he told anyone about these transactions. When all of this information becomes known to the patient's physician, the patient is asked to leave the hospital immediately. Despite the fact that the patient's infective endocarditis has not been treated optimally, he was discharged from the hospital against his will.

COMMENT. Considerations leading to an ethical justification of this decision are:

(a) *Medical indication.* The patient's use of intravenous street drugs at the same time that his physicians were attempting to eradicate his infective endocarditis indicated that the likelihood of medical success in this case, both short-term and long-term, was not great. Physicians are not obligated to treat people who simultaneously persist in actions that run directly counter to the goals of such treatment.

(b) *Patient wishes.* The patient preferred to be treated and, at the same time, to carry on his abusive and illegal behavior. The physicians are obliged to determine that the patient is competent to make such choices and that he was not suffering from a metabolic encephalopathy [2.2.3]. On the other hand, the physicians are not obliged to deal with the patient's long-standing sociopathic behavior pattern.

(c) *Interests of other patients.* This patient's physicians (who were hospital-based) had obligations both to this patient and to their other hospitalized patients. This patient's behavior of selling narcotics to other inpatients and of terrorizing his roommate compromised the care other patients of the same physician were receiving. This patient, then, posed a direct and serious threat to other identifiable persons [4.5.4].

(d) *Institutional needs.* The institution must provide appropriate care for all of its admitted patients. By his actions of striking nurses and of arguing with doctors and of terrorizing other patients, this patient was undermining the ability of the hospital to carry out its responsibilities to other patients. (See Chapter 4.)

2.8.3 **The Problem Patient: Socially Unacceptable.** Our reasoning in this case does not apply to most patients who present with critical illnesses, even for those illnesses for which the patient might be held responsible.

EXAMPLE. A 35-year-old chronic alcoholic with a long criminal record had emergency portacaval shunt for variceal bleeding. He continues to drink alcohol. Two years later, he presents twice within three months with acute bleeding from esophageal varices.

COUNSEL. This patient should be managed with aggressive medical and surgical means in an effort to control his hemorrhage and to reverse his blood loss. It takes more than past behavior to warrant physicians' withdrawing from the treatment of serious illness; indeed, the patient's past history should be ignored in most cases except insofar as it is medically relevant. Rather, refusal to treat a patient can be ethically justified in view of a person's behavior in the present circumstances when that behavior makes achievement of medical goals impossible [as in 2.8.2].

COMMENT. The problem with this patient is twofold. First, there is the suspicion that he will appear again, in the near future, with the same problem. Second, his problem was caused by personal behavior which is socially unacceptable, as is his style of life. The first problem raises the issues in Chapter 4 about allocation of scarce resources [4.5]; when the patient does become a repeater, the considerations mentioned there are relevant to a decision about his treatment. The second problem is discussed in Chapter 3, "Quality of Life." It should be noted that some harmful personal habits are more socially unacceptable than others. Substance abuse is strongly disapproved, while smoking, overeating, fast driving, not wearing seat belts, or engaging in dangerous sports are tolerated or even praised. Many conditions requiring expensive medical treatment are caused by behaviors that are socially accepted. Thus, singling out socially disapproved behaviors as less deserving of treatment reflects social prejudices rather than logic.

2.8.4 **Signing Out Against Medical Advice.** Mr. R. A., the patient described in 2.8.2, might leave the hospital before physicians judge his treatment adequate. When patients do discharge themselves in this manner, most hospitals request them to sign a statement confirming that they are leaving against medical advice (AMA). Of course, the patient cannot be forced to sign the statement; they have the right to leave at will. The document merely provides legal evidence of the fact of the patient's voluntary departure and warning by the physician of the risks of leaving. This warning, carried out as patiently and carefully as possible, is the ethical duty of the physician.

2.9 EDUCATION, PERSUASION, AND COERCION

The cases presented in 2.8–2.8.3 illustrate some issues of education, persuasion, and coercion that are applicable to ethical problems encountered in the COPE model. It is the obligation of the physician to educate patients about the best means for ameliorating their illness. It is the obligation of physicians to try to persuade patients to follow a course designed to achieve these goals. The physician's expertise often enables him/her to know more about the disease and its probable outcome than a patient knows. However, coercion is ethically unacceptable (conceding the line between persuasion and coercion may at times be blurred). Physicians should not engage in deception to trick patients into compliance. In 2.8.2 the disruptive patient clearly is beyond persuasion. The coercive acts of threatening him with expulsion and then forcing him to leave the hospital are justified only by his own coercive acts against others. (EB: BEHAVIOR CONTROL; BEHAVIORAL THERAPIES; FREE WILL AND DETERMINISM.)

2.9.1 **Withdrawing from Case.** At times, in COPE situations that are not working out well, the physician may serve the patient best by deciding to dissolve the physician–patient relationship and by helping the patient to find another physician. As we noted in 1.1.3, the physician's principal goal is to help the patient in the care of his or her health. If, for whatever reasons, this proves impossible, the physician may best demonstrate clinical discretion by withdrawing from the case and by finding another physician who might be more successful with the patient in these particular circumstances.

2.10 ABANDONMENT

Physicians who terminate the relationship with a patient sometimes wonder whether they can be charged with "abandonment." A legal definition of abandonment is "the unilateral severance by the physician of the professional relationship between himself and a patient without reasonable notice, at a time when there is still the necessity of continued medical attention" (McIntyre, 1962). Charges of abandonment can arise when the physician simply ceases to care for the patient without notice or when the physician is dilatory and careless (e.g., failing to visit the patient in the hospital or failing to judge the patient's condition serious enough to warrant attention). A charge of abandonment can usually be countered by showing that the patient did receive warning in sufficient time to arrange for medical care. There is no legal obligation on the physician to arrange for further care from another physician, although there is a legal obligation to provide full medical records to the new attending physician. If the physician does intend to maintain the relationship with the patient but will be unavailable for a time, there is a legal obligation to arrange for coverage by another physician. Failure to do so can be construed as abandonment.

Even though legal requirements have been met, a physician may be ethically blamed for abandoning a patient. If the patient is in serious need of care and has no other recourse, the physician has an ethical obligation to continue, despite provocation. That obligation is, of course, limited by several conditions. If the patient absorbs excessive time and energy, creating risk to other patients, if the patient is acting in ways to frustrate the attainable medical goals, or if the patient is endangering others by overt action, any ethical obligation to continue care would be diminished. These conditions appear to be verified in 2.8.2.

2.10.1 **Conscientious Objection by the Physician.** Physicians have their own moral values. Patients may express preferences that the physician finds morally objectionable. Traditionally, medical ethics has required them to abstain from moral judgments about their patients in regard to medical care. *Examples:* An emergency room physician is expected to provide competent care to the wounded assailant of an elderly person as well as to the assaulted party; a physician should treat, without censure, venereal disease contracted in what the physician considers an immoral liaison.

On occasion physicians may be asked not merely to tolerate an immoral action but to participate in effecting an immoral action desired by the patient. *Examples:* A male patient requests a physician who considers transexualism morally wrong to prescribe female estrogens in order to promote secondary female sexual characteristics; a Catholic physician is asked to perform an abortion.

Physicians may refuse to cooperate in actions they judge immoral on grounds of conscience. It is important, in forming one's conscience, to separate the moral values to which one is committed from personal distaste or prejudice. *Example:* A physician refuses to undertake care of a Jehovah's Witness with a hemorrhagic diathesis "on moral grounds," while in fact the physician does not like to feel impotent or run the risk of "losing a patient."

Institutions and programs should establish policy about conscientious objection and make the policy clear to those who work in that institution or program. Physicians who avail themselves of this moral right should not be penalized or sanctioned. When the grounds for objection are not widely known, it is permissible to request the objector to explain publicly the reasons for conscientious objection and to examine these reasons in a fair and open way. *Examples:* A Catholic intern refuses to perform abortions during a rotation in OB/GYN. The reasoning behind this refusal is well known. The refusal should be honored. A physician drafted into the service requests early discharge because, "my dedication as a physician is incompatible with military service." This rationale is open to debate; superiors are ethically justified in asking the objector to defend the position in public.

Despite the appropriateness, on occasion, of a public defense of one's views, the sincerely held belief that some act is immoral should be honored. However, the tradition of conscientious objection has long maintained that states and organizations can dismiss or discipline the objector and the objector should accept this as the price of a clean conscience. Thus, a trainee in OB/GYN might be dismissed from a program for refusal to perform abortions (the program is obliged to make this clear to the applicant) or a military physician might be court-martialed. (EB: CIVIL DISOBEDIENCE IN HEALTH SERVICES.)

BIBLIOGRAPHY

2.0. *Autonomy*

Beauchamp, Childress. 1979: Chapter 3.*

Childress, J. F. Paternalism and Autonomy in Medical Decision Making. In Abernethy, 1980: 27.

Downie, R., Telfer, E. *Respect for Persons.* New York: Schocken, 1970.

Feinberg, J. *Social Philosophy.* Englewood Cliffs, N.J.: Prentice-Hall, 1973, Ch. 1,2,3,.

2.1. *Ethical, Legal, and Psychological Significance of Patient Preferences*

Brody, D. S. The Patient's Role in Clinical Decision Making. *Ann Intern Med,* 1980, **93:**718.

Cassell, E. J. The Healer's Art: A New Approach to the Doctor-Patient Relationship. Philadelphia: Lippincott, 1976.

Cousins, N. Anatomy of an Illness (as Perceived by the Patient). *N Engl J Med,* 1976, **295:**1458.

Duffy, D. L., Hamerman, D., Cohen, M. A. Communication Skills of House Officers. *Ann Intern Med,* 1980, **93:**354.

Eisenberg, J. M. Sociological Influences on Decision Making by Clinicans. *Ann Intern Med,* 1979, **90:**957.

Fiore, N. Fighting Cancer: One Patient's Perspective. *N Engl J Med,* 1979, **300:**284.

Winslade, W. J. Patient and Physician—Who is Responsible for What? *Contemp. Surg,* 1978, **13**:39.

Winslade, W. J. Contracts to Care. *Contemp. Surg.,* 1979, **14:**59.

2.1.3 *Physicians' Respect for Patient Preferences*

Fletcher, C. M. *Communication in Medicine.* Nuffield Provincial Hospitals Trust, 1973.

Henderson, L. J. Physician and Patient as a Social System. *N Engl J Med,* 1935, **212:**819.

* Complete citations for abbreviated references appear at the end of the book under "General References."

Korsch, B., Negrete, V. F. Doctor-Patient Communication. *Sci Amer,* 1974, **7**:66.

Kleinman, A., Eisenberg, L., Good, B. Culture, Illness and Care: Clinical Lessons from Anthropological and Cross Cultural Research. *Ann Intern Med,* 1978, **88**:251.

Masters, R. D. Is Contract an Adequate Basis for Medical Care? *Hastings Center Report,* 1975, **5**(6):24.

May, W. F. Code, Covenant, Contract or Philanthropy? *Hastings Center Report,* 1975, **5**(6):29.

Reiser, S. J. Words as Scalpels: Transmitting Evidence in the Clinical Dialogue. *Ann Intern Med,* 1980, **92**:837.

Sackett, D. L. Patients and Therapies: Getting the Two Together. *N Engl J Med,* 1978, **298**:278.

Siegler, M., Osmond, H. *Patienthood: The Art of Being a Responsible Patient.* New York: Macmillan, 1979

Szasz, T. S., Hollender, M. H. The Basic Models of the Doctor-Patient Relationship. *Arch Intern Med,* 1956, **97**:585. (In Gorovitz, 1976: 64.)

Veatch, R. M. Medical Ethics: Professional or Universal? *Harvard Theological Rev,* 1972, **65**:531. (In Gorovitz, 1976: 76.)

2.2 *Competency and Capacity to Choose*

Abernethy, V., Lundin, K. Competency and the Right to Refuse Medical Treatment. In Abernethy, 1980: 79.

Appelbaum, P. S., Roth, L. H. Clinical Issues in the Assessment of Competency. *Am J Psychiatr* (in press).

Golden, J. S., Johnston, G. D. Problems of Distortion in Doctor-Patient Relationships. *Psychiatry in Medicine,* 1970, **1**:127.

Jackson, D. L., Youngner, S. Patient Autonomy and 'Death With Dignity': Some Clinical Caveats. *N Engl J Med,* 1979, **301**:404.

Meisel, A., Roth, L. H., Lidz, C. W. Toward A Model of the Legal Doctrine of Informed Consent. *Am J Psychiatr,* 1977, **134**:285.

Robertson, J. A. Legal Norms and Procedures for Withholding Care from Incompetent Patients. In Abernethy, 1980: 99.

Roth, L. H., Meisel, A., Lidz, C. W. Tests of Competency to Consent to Treatment. *Am J Psychiatr,* 1977, **134**:279.

Wickler, D. Paternalism and the Mildly Retarded. *Phil Pub Affairs,* 1979, **8**:377.

2.3 *Informed Consent*

Alfidi, R. J. Informed Consent: A Study of Patient Reaction. *JAMA,* 1971, **216**:1325.

Alfidi, R. J. Controversy: Alternatives and Decisions in Complying with the Doctrine of Informed Consent. *Radiology,* 1975, **114**:231.

Almquist, N. J. When the Truth Can Hurt: Patient Mediated Informed Consent in Cancer Therapy. *UCLA-Alaska Law Rev,* 1980, **9**:201.

Annas, G. J. Informed Consent. *Ann Rev Med,* 1978, **29**:9.

Barber, B. *Informed Consent in Medical Therapy and Research.* New Brunswick, N. J.: Rutgers University Press, 1980.

Capron, A. M. Informed Consent in Catastrophic Disease Research and Treatment. University of Pennsylvania Law Rev. 1974; **123**:340.

Cassileth, B. R. et al. Informed Consent: Why Are Its Goals Imperfectly Realized? *N Engl J Med,* 1980, **302**:896.

Cassileth, B. R. et al. Information and Participation Preferences Among Cancer Patients. *Ann Intern Med,* 1980, **92**:832.

Donagan, A. Informed Consent in Therapy and Experimentation. *J Med Phil,* 1977, **2**:307.

Faden, R. R., Beauchamp, T. L. Informed Consent and Decision Making: The Impact of Disclosed Information. *Social Indicators Research,* 1980, **7**:313.

Faden, A. L., Faden, R. R. Informed Consent in Medical Practice with Particular Reference to Neurology. *Arch Neurol,* 1978, 35:761.

Freedman, B. A Moral Theory of Informed Consent. *Hastings Center Report,* 1975, **5**(4):32.

Katz, J. Informed Consent—A Fairy Tale? Law's Vision. *University of Pittsburgh Law Rev,* 1977, **39**:137.

Meisel, A., Kabnick, L. Informed Consent to Medical Treatment: An Analysis of Recent Legislation. *University of Pittsburgh Law Rev,* 1980, **41**:407.

Miller, L. J. Informed Consent I–IV. *JAMA,* 1980, **244**:2100, 2347, 2556.

Rosoff, A. Informed Consent: A Guide for Health Care Providers. Rockville, Md.: Aspen Systems Corp, 1981.

Smith, C. Therapeutic Privilege to Withhold Specific Diagnosis from Patients Sick with Serious or Fatal Disease. *Tennessee Law Rev,* 1946, **19**:349.

Walz, J. F., Scheuneman, T. W. Informed Consent to Therapy. *Northwestern Law Rev,* 1970, **64**:628.

2.4 *Truthful Disclosure*

Adler, H. M., Mammett, V. O. The Doctor-Patient Relationship Revisited: An Analysis of the Placebo Effect. *Ann Intern Med,* 1973, **78**:595.

Agich, G. J. When Consent Is Unbearable: An Alternative Case Approach. *J Med Ethics,* 1979, **5**:26.

Beauchamp, T., Childress, J. 1979: 202–209.

Benson, H., Epstein, M. The Placebo Effect: A Neglected Asset in Care of Patients. *JAMA,* 1975, **232**:1225.

Bok, S. The Ethics of Giving Placebos. *Sci Am,* 1974, **231**(5):17. (In Reiser, Dyke, Curran, 1977: 248; in Shannon, 1976: 255.)
Bok, S. *Lying: Moral Choice in Public and Private Life.* New York: Pantheon Books, 1978.
Brody, H. *Placebos and the Philosophy of Medicine.* Chicago: University of Chicago Press, 1980.
Cabot, R. C. The Use of Truth and Falsity in Medicine. *American Medicine,* 1903, **5**:344. (In Reiser, Dyke, Curran, 1977: 213.)
Cousins, N. A Layman Looks at Truthtelling in Medicine. *JAMA,* 1980, **244**:1929.
Goodwin, J. S., Goodwin, J. M., Vogel, A. U. Knowledge and Use of Placebos by Nurses and House Officers. *Ann Intern Med,* 1979, **91**:111.
Green, M. What Is Wrong with Placebos? *Values and Ethics in Health Care,* 1981 (in press).
Houston, W. R. The Doctor Himself as Therapeutic Agent. *Ann Intern Med,* 1938, **11**:1416.
Kottow, M. When Consent Is Unbearable. *J Med Ethics,* 1978, **4**:78.
Leslie, A. Ethics and the Practice of Placebo Therapy. *Am J Med,* 1954, **16**:854. (In Reiser, Dyke, Curran, 1977: 240).
Melmon, K. L., Morrelli, H. F. *Clinical Pharmacology.* 2nd ed. New York: Macmillan, 1978, Ch. 24.
Novack, D. H., et al. Changes in Physicians' Attitudes Toward Telling the Cancer Patient. *JAMA,* 1979, **241**:897–900.
Oken, D. What to Tell Cancer Patients: A Study of Medical Attitudes. *JAMA,* 1961, **175**:1120.
Shapiro, A. K. Factors Contributing to the Placebo Effect. *Am J Psychother,* 1964, **18**(Suppl 1):73.
Shapiro, A. K. The Placebo Effect in the History of Medical Treatment. *Am J Psychiat,* 1959, **116**:248.
Siegler, M. Pascal's Wager and the Hanging of Crepe. *N Engl J Med,* 1975, **293**:853.
Silber, T. J. Placebo Therapy: Ethical Dimension. *JAMA,* 1979, **242**:245.
Simmons, B. Problems in Deceptive Medical Procedures: An Ethical and Legal Analysis of Administration of Placebos. *J Med Ethics,* 1978, 4:172.
Veatch, R. M. 1976: Ch. 6.
Wells, F. The Moral Choice in Prescribing Barbiturates. *J Med Ethics,* 1976, **2**:68.

2.5 *Refusal of Treatment by Persons Competent to Choose*

Beauchamp, Childress. 1979: 163–164.
Buchanan, A. Medical Paternalism. *Phil Pub Affairs,* 1977, **7**:370.

Byrn, R. Compulsory Lifesaving Treatment for Competent Adults. *Fordham Law Rev,* 1975, **44**:1. (In Beauchamp, Walters, 1978: 150.)

Childress, J. F. Paternalism in Health Care. In Robison, Pritchard, 1979: 15.

Clinicosociologic Conferences: Decisions Regarding the Provision or Withholding of Therapy. *Am J Med,* 1976, **61**:915.

Dworkin, G. Paternalism. *The Monist,* 1972, **56**:64. (In Gorovitz, 1976: 185.)

Faden, R., Faden, A. False Belief and the Refusal of Medical Treatment. *J Med Ethics,* 1977, **3**:133.

Ford, J. Refusal of Blood Transfusions by Jehovah's Witnesses. *Catholic Lawyer,* 1964, **10**:212.

Gert, B., Culver, C. Paternalistic Behavior. *Phil Pub Affairs,* 1976, **6**:45. (In Robinson, Pritchard, 1979: 15.)

Hegland, K. F. Unauthorized Rendition of Life-Saving Medical Treatment. *California Law Rev,* 1965, **53**:860.

Jonas, H. The Right to Die. *Hastings Center Report,* 1978, **8**(4):31.

Lo, B., Jonsen, A. R. Ethical Decisions in the Care of a Patient Terminally Ill with Metastatic Cancer. *Ann Intern Med,* 1980, **92**:107.

McCartney, J. R. Refusal of Treatment: Suicide or Competent Choice? *Gen Hosp Psychiatr,* 1979, **1**:338.

McKegney, F. P., Lange, P. The Decision to No Longer Live on Chronic Dialysis. *Am J Psychiatr,* 1971, **128**:47.

Macklin, R. Consent, Coercion and Conflict of Rights. *Perspect Biol Med,* 1977, **20**:360.

Marsh, F. H. An Ethical Approach to Paternalism in the Patient Physician Relationship. *Ethics Sci Med,* 1977, **4**:135.

Paris, J. J. Compulsory Medical Treatment and Religious Freedom: Whose Law Shall Prevail? *University of San Francisco Law Rev,* 1975, **10**:1.

Perry, C. Paternalism as a Supererogatory Act. *Ethics Sci Med* 1979, **6**:155.

Siegler, M. Critical Illness: The Limits of Autonomy. *Hastings Center Report,* 1977, **7**(5):12.

Veatch, R. M. 1976: Ch. 4.

2.6 *The Living Will*

Bok, S. Personal Directions for Care at the End of Life. *N Engl J Med,* 1976, **295**:367.

Jonsen, A. R. Dying Right in California: The California Natural Death Act. *Clin Research,* 1978, **26**:55.

Kaplan, P. R. Euthanasia Legislation. *Am J Law Med,* 1976, **2**:41.

Lappe, M. Dying While Living: A Critique of Allowing to Die Legislation. *J Med Ethics,* 1978, **4**:195.

Veatch, R. M. Death and Dying: The Legislative Options. *Hastings Center Report,* 1977, **7**(5):5.

Winslade, W. J. Thoughts on Technology and Death: An Appraisal of California's Natural Death Act. *DePaul Law* Rev 1977, **26:**717.

2.6.1 *Extraordinary and Ordinary Measures*

Ashley, B. M., O'Rourke, K. D. 1978: 387.

Kelly, G. *Medico Moral Problems.* St. Louis: Catholic Hospital Assn, 1958, Ch. 17.

McCartney, J. J. The Development of the Doctrine of Ordinary and Extraordinary Means of Preserving Life in Catholic Moral Theology Before the Karen Quinlan Case. *Linacre Q,* 1980, **47:**215.

O'Neil, R. In Defense of the Ordinary-Extraordinary Distinction. *Linacre Q,* 1978, **45:**37.

Ramsey, P. 1970: Ch. 3.

Veatch, R. M. 1976: Ch. 3.

2.7.1 *Implied Consent*

Tait, K. M., Winslow, G. Beyond Consent: The Ethics of Decision Making in Emergency Medicine. *West J Med,* 1977, **126:**156.

2.7.3 *Consent of Minors*

Ackerman, T. F. The Limits of Beneficence: Jehovah's Witnesses and Childhood Cancer. *Hastings Center Report,* 1980, **10**(4):13.

Hoffman, A. A Rational Policy Toward Consent and Confidentiality in Adolescent Health Care. *J Adolescent Med,* 1980, **1:**9.

Holder, A. *Legal Issues in Pediatrics and Adolescent Medicine.* New York: John Wiley, 1977.

Petschesky, P. R. Reproduction, Ethics, and Public Policy: Federal Sterilization Regulations. *Hastings Center Report,* 1979, **9**(5):29.

Showalter, J. E., et al. The Adolescent Patient's Decision to Die. Pediatr, 1973, **51:**97. (In Gorovitz, 1976: 414.)

2.8 *Failure to Comply with Medical Regimen*

Bissonette, R., Seller, R. Medical Noncompliance: A Cultural Perspective. *Man and Medicine,* 1980, **5:**42.

Gaylin, W. On The Borders of Persuasion: A Psychoanalytic Look at Coercion. *Psychiatry,* 1974, **37:**1.

Groves, J. E. Taking Care of the Hateful Patient. *N Engl J Med,* 1978, **297:**883.

Haynes, L. B., Taylor, D. W., Sackett, D. C. *Compliance in Health Care.* Baltimore: The Johns Hopkins Press, 1979.

Meenan, R. F. Improving the Public's Health: Some Further Reflections. *N Engl J Med,* 1976, **294:**45.

Sackett, D. L., Haynes, R. B. (eds.). *Compliance with Therapeutic Regimens*. Baltimore: Johns Hopkins Press, 1976.

Veatch, R. M. Voluntary Risks to Health. *JAMA,* 1980, **243**:50.

Wickler, D. Persuasion and Coercion for Health: Ethical Issues in Government Efforts to Change Life Styles. *Health and Society—Milbank Mem Q.*, 1978, **56**:303.

Winterbottom, S. Coping with the Violent Patient in Accident and Emergency. *J Med Ethics,* 1979, **5**:124.

2.10 *Abandonment*

Holder, A. *Medical Malpractice Law*. New York: John Wiley & Sons, 1975, 357.

McIntyre, L. L. The Action of Abandonment in Medical Malpractice Litigation. *Tulane Law Rev,* 1962, **36**:834.

Cassel, C. K., Jameton, A. L. Dementia in the Elderly: An analysis of medical responsibility. *Ann Intern Med,* 1981, **94**:802–807.

2.10.1 *Conscientious Objection by the Physician*

Ashley, O'Rourke. 1979: 197.

Curran, C. E. Cooperation: Toward a Revision of the Concept. *Linacre Q.,* 1974, **41**:152.

Childress, J. *Civil Disobedience and Political Obligation*. New Haven: Yale University Press, 1971.

Siegler, M. Searching for Moral Certainty in Medicine: A Proposal for a New Model of the Doctor-Patient Encounter. *Bull NY Acad Med,* 1981, **57**:56.

3

QUALITY OF LIFE

3.0 This chapter concerns quality of life insofar as that subject influences clinical ethical decisions. It discusses (a) the meaning of this phrase in clinical ethical deliberations; (b) the use of quality-of-life judgments in decisions to terminate or withhold therapy; (c) the related concept of "quality of death" in discussions of euthanasia; (d) use of pain medication for dying persons; and (e) suicide.

The competent practice of medicine should aspire to improve the quality of life of patients. The goals of medicine envision this improvement in quality of life: restoration of health, relief of pain and symptoms, and support of compromised function. The fifteenth-century medical maxim "cure occasionally, relieve frequently, comfort always" implies these goals. There is little question about medicine's dedication to enhancing quality of life, but there are many questions about what quality of life consists of, about who determines quality of life, and about the effects of such judgments on the care provided to the patient.

The ethical principles underlying the considerations in this chapter are complex. Considerations of quality of life enter into decisions to act in accord with the principle of beneficence, that is, to do good and avoid harm. These considerations also arise in the utilitarian form of ethical deliberation, which involves, in part, the intention to effect a greater balance of pleasure over pain in the experiences of a person, of a population, or in the world. (EB: ETHICS; UTILITARIANISM.)

3.1 CLINICAL ETHICAL DELIBERATIONS

The phrase "quality of life" is now frequently heard in clinical discussions about ethical problems. Frequent use has given the phrase neither any precise meaning nor any definite application. It seems to represent an attempt to put a value upon some feature, or collection of features, of human experience. As such, it is highly subjective; yet the phrase is often used by someone other than the person who is living the life being evaluated. Also, the phrase is used as if there were certain objective criteria, even though, as an evaluation, it rests less on facts than upon preferences about those facts. The following cases reveal the ambiguity hidden in the phrase "quality of life." (EB: LIFE; QUALITY OF LIFE; VALUE OF LIFE.)

3.1.1 Clinical Examples.

EXAMPLE I. A 23-year-old gymnastics instructor suffers a spinal cord lesion at C2-C3 level. He is alert and oriented.

EXAMPLE II. A 68-year-old artist suffers from chronic diabetes mellitus and now faces blindness and multiple amputations. She is in renal failure.

EXAMPLE III. A 37-year-old chronic alcoholic suffers 60 percent total body burns.

EXAMPLE IV. A 29-year-old retarded man with an IQ of 20 and mental age of three years is difficult to manage and keep clean, and frequently hurts himself.

EXAMPLE V. An 82-year-old woman resident of a nursing home has advanced senile dementia.

EXAMPLE VI. A 42-year-old police officer is in extreme pain with cancer of the pancreas.

EXAMPLE VII. A 27-year-old woman, recently divorced and having lost her job, is suffering from extreme depression.

COMMENT. Someone, whether the sufferer or an observer, might say about any of these cases, "What a terrible life!" (equivalently, a life of poor quality). What might such a comment mean?

(a) It might mean, in general, that the sufferer's experiences fall below some standard that the speaker considers desirable. But in each case the experience in question is different; it can be pain (the standard being a pain-free existence), loss of mobility, presence of multiple debilitating health problems, loss of mental capacity and of the enjoyment of human interaction, loss of joy in life, and so on. Poor quality of life, then, refers to many quite different circumstances.

(b) The judgment of poor quality of life may be made by the one who lives the life or by an observer. It often happens that lives which observers consider of poor quality are lived quite satisfactorily by the one living that life. Human beings are amazingly adaptable. They can make the best of the options available. For example, the quadriplegic gymnastics instructor may be a person of extraordinary motivation; the blind artist may enjoy a vivid imagination; the retarded person may experience simple pleasures.

(c) Evaluation of the quality of life, like life itself, changes over time. The depressed woman may soon be vital or may be more depressed; the cancer patient may be rendered pain-free by skillful use of analgesics or be subject to intractable pain.

"Quality of life," then, has a variety of uses. Yet the term often appears in medical literature and in clinical discussions as if it could be used in a simple, unequivocal way. Thus, physicians should be vividly aware of the variety of uses and the possibility for ambiguity. When the term is introduced into a discussion, several questions should be asked: Who is making the evaluation? What aspect of life is under consideration? What measure or criterion is being used? What are the possibilities for change in the objective condition? In particular, it is crucial to make explicit the biases of those making the judgment.

3.1.2 **Discussion in the Clinical Setting.** In the clinical setting, discussion about a patient's quality of life can take many forms. *Example:* Physicians, nurses, and social workers may discuss living conditions, pain relief, and problems of mobility in view of alleviating the poor quality of life for an elderly person with severe arthritis. *Example:* Physicians and nurses may discuss a suitable pain-medication regimen for the patient with cancer of the pancreas, attempting to achieve maximum relief together with minimal loss of consciousness and of communication with family. This sort of discussion poses no ethical problem; indeed, it should be a part of any therapeutic plan.

3.1.3 **Definition.** "Quality of life" is a phrase that does not lend itself to satisfactory definition. Still, common use seems to support the following definitions. The primary definition is:

(a) Quality of life may refer to the subjective satisfaction expressed or experienced by an individual in his physical, mental, and social situation (even though these may be deficient in some manner). *Example:* The gymnastics instructor [3.1.1] states, "The quality of my life is excellent, though, to see me, you wouldn't believe it. I've come to terms with my loss and discovered the powers of my mind."

Two secondary definitions are:

(b) Quality of life refers to the objective achievement by certain persons of attributes and skills that are highly valued in our culture, e.g., intellectual ability, physical capacity, emotional stability, artistic and technical skills, capacity to form and enjoy social relationships. The criteria are, of course, various and differently ranked in importance.

(c) Quality of life may refer to the subjective evaluation by an onlooker of another's subjective experiences of personal life. *Examples:* The nurse describes the pain of the cancer patient, "Pain is all-consuming. His life simply has no quality at all."

Speaking of the elderly woman in the nursing home, her daughter says, "She used to be so vital. Now the quality of her life is just terrible."

NOTE. The phrase "quality of life" may not actually be used in such discussions. Other terms express the same intent, namely, a judgment of relative value experienced in one's own life or presumed about another's experiences. Often the issue is latent and implicit in a discussion. *Example:* The doctor says that workup of the elderly woman's fever "wouldn't do much good." Implicit in this statement is the judgment that the quality of the person's life would not improve even if the cause of fever were found and successfully treated. The statement is shorthand for "she would be better off dead."

.1.4 **Grading.** Although such adjectives as "high" and "low," "acceptable" and "unacceptable" are used to describe quality of life, such grading is very problematic. If a person says his own life is "acceptable," the standards are his own; if an onlooker says of another's life, "it is unacceptable," the standards are those of the onlooker, who *presumes* the other would not find a life of that sort acceptable. Further, given the many elements that might make a life satisfactory to an individual, it seems impossible to find common measures or scales for grading. However, some human situations do seem so bad that they would be universally rejected. No one would choose them if the choice were offered. Those who suffer them do so unwillingly or must summon up the greatest heroism. Extreme physical pain, deterioration of motor capacities and loss of control over one's body, profound impairment of mental functioning, incessant and deep emotional turmoil are a few of the human situations that might, with some justification, be evaluated as contributing to lessened or low quality of life.

.1.5 **Subjective Evaluation by Onlooker.** Among the many meanings and uses of the phrase "quality of life," we choose to use the phrase to refer to *subjective evaluation by an onlooker about another's life, when the other is unable to make such an evaluation or express it because of mental incapacity.* We select this usage because it is the one that usually seems to be at issue in crucial ethical deliberations about patient care. In this book "*poor quality*" refers to the existence of severe deficits of physical health, mental health, or social interaction. The phrase "*minimal quality*" refers to situations in which general physical condition has deteriorated beyond recovery and in which interaction between the patient and others is severely restricted. The phrase "*below the threshold considered minimal*" refers to extreme physical debilitation and a complete loss of sensory and intellectual activity. *Note:* Making these distinctions and referring them to some very general clinical situations *implies nothing* about how these distinctions should be used as justifications for decisions. Use of these distinctions is discussed in the following paragraphs.

3.2 QUALITY OF LIFE AND TERMINATION OF LIFE SUPPORT

Quality-of-life discussions often take place in situations where an ethical decision must be made about continuing life-supporting interventions. *These situations involve a patient who is not able to express personal preferences at all or whose expression is indiscernible or indecipherable as a result of illness and whose physical condition is critical. In addition, physicians suspect that, if some suggested intervention succeeds, the patient will survive, but with severe deficits of physical or mental capacity*. The question then is asked, "Is such a life worth living?" In this sense, raising the issue of quality of life seems equivalent to wondering whether no life at all is better than a life with certain deficits. This is a metaphysical question, but physicians faced with such decisions seldom enjoy the leisure for metaphysical speculation. The following sections suggest some considerations appropriate to clinical decisions of this sort.

CASE I. Mr. CARE (CARE model 1.4) suffering from advanced multiple sclerosis, has a respiratory arrest associated with gram-negative pneumonia and septicemia. He is placed on a respirator. Within one week a neurology consultant states that Mr. CARE has the neurological signs consistent with chronic vegetative state. At no time in the course of his care has he expressed any clear preferences about his future. Should respirator support be continued?

COMMENT. (a) Mr. CARE is not brain dead in the strict sense of having lost all function of both higher and lower brain. He still has brain stem activity, respiration, and heartbeat. Thus, he is not legally dead [1.7].

(b) Medical interventions promise no benefit beyond sustaining organic life [1.5].

(c) All the functions usual to human interaction and, to the best of the observer's knowledge, all forms of cognitive and sensory experience are absent or extremely deficient. It is extremely unlikely that any of these functions will be recovered.

(d) Note how this case differs from 1.4.4(d), in which Mr. CARE is dead according to brain criteria, and 1.4.4(a), in which his death is imminent. In those situations the judgment that further intervention is entirely useless, in terms of achieving medical goals, justifies the decision to discontinue mechanical support. In this case Mr. CARE is neither dead nor imminently dying. If respirator support is continued, he will not recover from his disease, nor will he return to mental functioning sufficient for communication. His life, supported by mechanical means, will consist of vegetative activities alone (as far as anyone knows). On the other hand, if respirator support is removed, Mr. CARE may breathe on his own and continue to live in persistent vegetative state. Life in a vegetative state seems to the physician and the family a life of low—indeed, of no—quality. Their expectation is that, once the respirator is discontinued, Mr. CARE will die quickly as the result of his fatal and long disease. [Cf. 1.7.1–1.7.2 on "Clinical Signs of Persistent Vegetative State."]

COUNSEL. In our judgment it is ethically permissible to discontinue life support. We argue that the conjunction of three features of this case justifies such a decision. (1) We propose that the state of an irreversible loss of human cognitive and communicative function implies that a "person" no longer exists in any significant sense of the term. This individual is no longer aware of self in relation to surroundings and never will be again. In our terms life has fallen irretrievably below the threshold considered minimal. (2) As a result, no goals of medicine other than support of organic life are being or will be accomplished. We do not believe this goal, in and of itself, is an independent and overriding goal of medicine. (3) No preferences of the patient are expressed or known. The conjunction of these three factors justifies, in our judgment, a decision not to continue medical intervention—that is, physicians have no ethical obligation to continue treatment (nor do they have any ethical *obligation* to *discontinue,* unless other considerations, such as patient preferences [Chapter 2] and external factors [Chapter 4] become decisive). The same argument does not, in and of itself, justify active euthanasia. This is a more complicated question discussed under the heading "Euthanasia" [3.3].

> CASE II. Mr. CARE is in the same condition as described above in Case I. However, he is not on a respirator. He now becomes anuric and is in renal failure. Should dialysis be initiated?

COMMENT. There is no significant ethical difference between Case I and Case II; from the point of view of medical goals, of patient preference, and of assessment of quality of life, the situation is the same. This version, however, involves an instance of not starting an intervention rather than stopping one already being used. Many interventions are initiated at times when their use is quite rational: The achievement of important goals is still seen as possible. When these goals cannot be achieved, and when there are other important considerations, e.g., absence of patient preference and quality of life below the minimal threshold, they may be discontinued. In other situations the question is raised whether to initiate another intervention, in face of a new problem, or as a "last ditch stand." *It is our position that there is no significant ethical difference between stopping and starting, if the essential considerations regarding medical indications, patient preference, and quality of life are the same.*

There may be a psychological or emotional difference: Some physicians find it more troubling to stop an ongoing intervention than not to initiate a new one. The initiation of treatment expresses some measure of optimism. If, despite the physician's efforts, the patient succumbs to the disease, the physician has tried and done his best. However, in withdrawing or stopping treatment, a decision motivated by loss of hope, the physician concedes defeat. In stopping life-supporting treatment, the therapeutic relationship is being severed irrevocably. The physician becomes responsible (in a causal sense) for the events that follow, even though he may bear no responsibility (in the sense of ethical or legal accountability) either for the disease process or for the patient's succumbing to the disease.

Finally, after deciding to refrain from aggressive therapeutic efforts, new medical problems, such as infection or renal failure, sometimes tempt physicians to initiate therapeutic interventions to deal with these particular problems. This is, of course, irrational, unless the intervention has as its purpose another goal more appropriate to the situation, such as providing comfort to the dying patient [cf. 1.6.4; 3.4].

3.2.1 **Legal Implications.** The death of a patient resulting from a decision to discontinue medical intervention on the grounds mentioned in 3.2 ("Counsel") has legal implications. In the cases described in that section, the patient could be kept alive, perhaps for some time, by continued use of the respirator, by dialysis, or in some other way. It is the "quality" of that continued life that leads to the decision to cease intervention. In contrast, the cases mentioned in 1.5 involved persons whose death was imminent and for whom further intervention was judged useless in terms of medical goals. These latter cases are not likely to generate legal problems unless someone, such as a relative or another physician, claims the judgment of medical uselessness was wrongly made or not made with due care. The former cases, namely those where quality of life is the central issue, are more legally problematic: A person who *could* be kept alive is allowed to die. In legal theory this might be considered homicide (although the traditional definitions of homicide certainly did not envision the problems occasioned by modern medical technology). The physician might be accused of criminal negligence or named as an accomplice in the illegal decision of another if he accedes to or does not object to the discontinuing of life support by another. These are theoretical possibilities. To our knowledge no physician has been criminally prosecuted in cases of this sort. Nevertheless, fear of these theoretical possibilities, coupled with conservative legal advice, often causes physicians to hesitate in making decisions of this sort. However, in several important legal cases, courts have given approval to decisions to withhold or terminate life support. The Karen Ann Quinlan case was the first of these. The legal arguments in these cases are complex and controversial. Although the courts have been reluctant to base decisions on "quality-of-life" grounds, the legal perplexities are being resolved to some extent.

COUNSEL. In cases of this sort, it is our opinion that physicians are acting within the law, as currently understood, when they decide to withhold or withdraw life-supporting interventions. The conditions required for this decision are: (1) It is virtually certain that further medical intervention will not attain any of the goals of medicine other than sustaining organic life; (2) the preferences of the patient are not known and cannot be expressed; (3) quality of life clearly falls below the threshold considered minimal; (4) family and members of the staff are in accord. We hold this opinion because, despite the legal perplexities, the leading cases thus far adjudicated have affirmed the legal correctness of allowing the patient to die when these conditions are present. In addition, we consider it advisable for institutions to establish an appropriate review committee for cases that present problems, particularly regarding medical indications [cf. 4.1.6]. Finally, institutions should request their legal counsels to prepare clear instructions for the medical staff in view of prevailing local law.

3.2.2. **Judicial Decisions.** The most important judicial decisions relevant to cases of this sort are summarized in Table IV. These summaries are very brief and, given the legal complexities, may be misleading. They are here stated only to familiarize the reader with the names of the cases and the principal issue. Fuller information can be found by consulting the articles referenced at 3.2.1.

3.2.3 **Poor Quality of Life.** In the above cases [3.2] Mr. CARE's condition, a persistent vegetative state, represents a quality of life falling below what we have called the "threshold considered minimal." In such situations, the ethical justification for refrain-

Table IV. JUDICIAL DECISIONS RELATING TO LIFE-SUPPORTING INTERVENTIONS

In the Matter of Shirley Dinnerstein, 380 N.E.2d 134 (Mass. Appeals Ct 1978) [upheld validity of "no-code" order on 67-year-old woman suffering from Alzheimer's disease and ruled that such orders did not need court approval].

Application of Eichner [*Fox*], 426 N.Y.S.2d 517 (decision of New York Supreme Court Appellate Division, Second Judicial Dept, decided March 27, 1980), affirming 423 N.Y.S.2d 580 (Supt Ct, Nassau County, Special Term, Part VI, 1979) [trial court authorized guardian of 83-year-old religious brother in "irreversible vegetative state" to request that respirator be discontinued, based on evidence of patient's prior wishes. Appellate court affirmed and laid out procedures to be followed in future cases].

Parker v. U.S., 406 A.2d 1275 (District of Columbia Ct of Appeals 1979) [in this criminal case, the defendant sought to overturn his conviction by claiming that discontinuance of life-support system on brain-damaged victim was the cause of her death. Defendant argued that any termination of "heroic measures" without a court order is always unreasonable. The Court affirmed the conviction, saying: "We reject that argument. No legal authority is cited or appears to exist that requires courts to intervene when extraordinary life support methods are threatened with withdrawal pursuant to a so-called 'living will' or as here (citing *Dinnerstein,* above)" (at page 1282)].

In re Quinlan, 355 A.2d 647 (N.J. Supreme Ct 1976) [authorized discontinuance of life-support system for 21-year-old comatose woman in permanent vegetative state, based on her constitutional right of privacy as asserted by her parents on her behalf. Required prior review by a hospital ethics committee.]

Superintendent of Belchertown State School v. Saikewicz, 370 N.E.2d 417 (Mass. Supreme Ct 1977) [affirmed trial court decision to not order chemotherapy on 67-year-old severely retarded and institutionalized man suffering from acute myeloblastic leukemia, also on right to privacy grounds, but stressed the role of courts in reviewing such questions].

In the Matter of Spring, 405 N.E.2d 115 (Mass. Sup. Jud. Ct 1980), reversing 399 N.E.2d 493 (Mass. Ct of Appeals 1979) and remanding the judgment to the trial court for further hearings) [upheld right of 77-year-old man (who subsequently died in April 1980 during these proceedings) who was senile and suffered from kidney disease to stop hemodialysis treatment. The Supreme Court emphasized that this was not a decision to be delegated to the attending physician, and the man's wife and son, but rather must be made by the probate court on appropriate findings].

ing from medical intervention seems to us quite strong. However, in other cases, quality of life, although an important consideration, is a more dubious ethical justification for a decision to refrain from intervention.

CASE I. Mr. B. B. is 94 years old and living in a nursing home. He sits all day in a chair, without responding to any human attention. He is difficult to feed, frequently choking and expelling food. He has been treated several times in the past month for aspiration pneumonia with antibiotics and fluids. During the night he develops a violent cough and wheezing. He has a fever of 100. The visiting physician diagnoses aspiration pneumonia. Should he be treated again? [1.4–1.4.4.]

CASE II. Mrs. A. W., a 44-year-old woman, married with three children, has had a long history of scleroderma and ischemic ulcerations of fingers and toes. She is admitted with signs of renal failure. The big toe of her right foot and several fingers of her left hand became gangrenous. Several days later she consents to amputation of the right foot and the thumb and first finger of her left hand. After surgery she is alternately obtunded and confused. She develops pneumonia and is placed on a respirator. The remaining fingers of her left hand become gangrenous and more extensive amputation is required. Her renal condition worsens, and it is now necessary to consider initiating dialysis. The attending says, "How could anyone want to live a life of such terrible quality?" Should the respirator be discontinued? Should dialysis be initiated? [1.4–1.4.4.]

COMMENT. In Mr. B. B.'s case, quality of life refers to the observers' assessment in view of low levels of physical and mental activity. Nothing is known about Mr. B. B.'s own subjective experience. Similarly, the severe physical deficits and the problems of rehabilitation faced by Mrs. A. W. evoke in the observer an assessment that "no one would want to live that way." This, of course, cannot be verified by Mrs. A. W. at this time. There is a difference that might be ethically relevant. Mr. B. B. will suffer recurring episodes of aspiration. Even tube feeding might not resolve this problem. Thus, after several episodes it is ethically permissible to refrain from treatment of pneumonia, permitting this disease to be, as it was once called, "the old man's friend." Quality of life, then, has become a relevant consideration, but only insofar as it refers to an objective state, particularly inability to control motor activities and to cooperate with care in any way. This objective state makes achievement of medical goals increasingly impossible at the same time medical problems continue to arise.

In contrast, Mrs. A. W. has multiple problems, but all are potentially reversible, with the exception of the loss of extremities. Achievement of significant medical goals is possible. In addition, she herself has consented to the initial amputations, suggesting her willingness to live with these deficits. Finally, her vital personality prior to her surgery suggested to the staff that she had the ability to cope with rehabilitation and the difficulties of subsequent life.

COUNSEL. In our opinion it is ethically permissible to refrain from treating Mr. B. B.'s pneumonia after several episodes have shown this to be the beginning of a recurring pattern. There is no obligation to proceed with measures such as gastrostomy or gastrogavage. On the other hand, it is ethically obligatory to continue to treat Mrs. A. W.

3.2.4 **Quality-of-Life Judgments and Mental Retardation or Mental Illness.** Quality-of-life judgments are sometimes made about persons whose lives are limited as a result of mental retardation or mental illness. Given the range of possibilities for social intercourse, intellectual achievement, personal accomplishment, and productivity open to most human beings, these persons seem severely restricted. It might be said, then, that they live a life of poor or low quality (in the sense of definitions b and c in 3.1.3). When decisions about medical care are made for such persons, is such quality of life a relevant consideration?

CASE III. Mr. A. S. is a 67-year-old man who has been institutionalized for mental retardation since the age of one. His mental age is estimated at less than the three-year-old level, and his IQ is 10. He develops acute nonlymphoblastic leukemia. His guardian says, "His life is such poor quality. Why should we try to extend it?" [1.3–1.3.3.]

COMMENT. The above case recalls an actual one in which an important legal decision was rendered (cf. Table IV). The court approved a decision not to treat Mr. Saikewicz with chemotherapy. However, the court attempted to distinguish between the quality of life of retarded persons, which it did not consider relevant to the decision, and the quality of life that Joseph Saikewicz "was likely to experience" under treatment. Speaking of the continued state of pain and disorientation likely to result from chemotherapy, the court said, "He would experience fear without the understanding from which other patients draw strength." This distinction suggests a point of great ethical importance. Deciding to withhold medical treatment from an individual because that individual belongs to a *class* of persons whose lives are limited in view of social norms for accomplishment and productivity is ethically perilous. It looks more to the burden these persons place on society than to the burden these persons might be to themselves. We usually do not know whether, and to what extent, these persons experience themselves as "burdensome" to themselves or experience their life as "of poor quality." On the other hand, we are aware of the burdens their existence places on others. This argument is discussed in Chapter 4. The *Saikewicz* court, like all courts that have dealt with such cases, wishes to avoid this argument. The court's reasoning is an attempt to rely on the autonomy of the patient (Chapter 2). It proposes a doctrine of "substituted judgment," suggesting we have good reason to assume that Mr. A. S., as an individual person, might prefer not to be treated if he experienced the adverse effects of chemotherapy without being able to understand why. In addition, the considerations of Chapter 1 are reflected in the judgment that the likelihood of remission in Mr. A. S.'s case is extremely low. Thus, the court tries to tailor the decision to Mr. A. S. as an individual and allows an assessment of the pain and suffering that he personally will experience to become a decisive consideration. The decision warns against considering Mr. A. S. merely as a member of a class of persons of "poor quality life." If poor quality of life is relevant, it is not the "poor quality" that observers see in the daily existence of a retarded person. It is the life of pain and suffering without understanding that A. S. will experience during chemotherapy (together with a low chance of remission) which constitutes poor quality. A peril of seeing persons as class members for the purpose of medical treatment is the "slippery slope," i.e., starting a process in which classes of "undesirables" grow increasingly wider and sweep in more and more persons who are "burdens to themselves and others." This argument is discussed in 3.3 under the heading "euthanasia."

3.2.5 **The Distasteful Patient.** There are persons in need of medical care whose manner of life and behavior are extremely distasteful to those who must care for them. They arouse quite negative feelings, which are often expressed in "quality-of-life" terms. True, from many points of view their lives are of "poor quality." Should quality-of-life judgments be relevant to decisions about their treatment? [Cf. 2.8.2–2.8.3.]

CASE IV. Mr. C. D. is an alcoholic who inhabits building excavations. He is extremely filthy, foul-mouthed, and, at times, violent and disruptive. He appears quite regularly at the hospital in need of various sorts of care for pneumonia, frostbite, delirium tremens, and so forth. One of the house officers, despite a reprimand from the chief resident, persists in calling him Gomer the Gopher. He is brought to the ER for the third time in a month with bleeding esophageal varices. The ER intern says, "High quality of life like C's we can do without." [1.3–1.3.3, 1.4–1.4.4.]

COMMENT. Mr. C. D.'s quality of life, while certainly low in terms of the objective values of our culture, is not relevant to medical decisions. The question of the burden he imposes on others may be relevant. This is considered in 2.8.2, 4.4, and 4.5.

3.2.6 **Conclusions.** (a) Quality of life may be considered as decisive in a clinical decision to withhold or withdraw interventions necessary for life when the following conditions are all present:

(i) The indications of medical treatment are such that the goal of preservation of organic life without attainment of the other goals is likely to be the only accomplishment, or the achievement of other medical goals capable of contributing to continued life is very unlikely [1.1.3–1.1.5].

(ii) The preferences of the patient are not and cannot be known [2.1–2.2.5].

(iii) The quality of life of the patient falls below the minimum threshold [3.1.5–3.2].

In cases where all these conditions are not fulfilled, poor quality of life should not be a decisive consideration. Indeed, it should be suspect; the sorts of judgments that healthy, intelligent, socially accomplished, and technically skilled persons make about the ill, incompetent, or uneducated and unskilled are very likely to be biased. In addition, differences of social and economic class can lead to widely different views of what constitutes a tolerable quality of life.

(b) In addition, the acceptance of quality of life as a criterion for treatment decisions can lead to undesirable social consequences. Judgments of good and bad quality may begin with quite generally accepted notions and be slowly enlarged and generalized. All sorts of "unacceptables" can be swept into the category of persons living lives of poor quality: hippies, gypsies, the uneducated and illiterate, persons of low intelligence or with physical handicaps, those of unfamiliar cultural backgrounds or racial origins disfavored by the majority, and so on. Persons adjudged to fall into these vague categories may no longer be seen as "deserving help."

(c) Medicine has an ancient ethical tradition of caring for all in need, regardless of social, racial, economic, or political identity. The Temple of the Healing God, Aesculapius, in Greece was inscribed:

> Physicians must be like gods:
> bringing benefit to all alike,
> the rich and the poor, men and
> women, friend and enemy.

Thus, quality-of-life considerations, although often relevant, sometimes important, and on quite specific occasions decisive, should be viewed very cautiously when invoked to justify an ethical decision about whether medical treatment should be provided.

3.3 EUTHANASIA

Quality of life and quality of death may be associated: Patients who are in severe pain during terminal disease certainly are living what would appear to be a life of poor quality. It may occur to them or to others that they would be "better off dead." Profound questions are asked: "Is it better to take measures to bring about a peaceful death than to continue in such a state?" The term "euthanasia," meaning "good death," sometimes appears in this context. (EB: DEATH AND DYING, EUTHANASIA AND SUSTAINING LIFE.)

3.3.1 **Definition.** The word "euthanasia" is used in many different ways, resulting in considerable confusion. In one sense, perhaps the popular sense, it refers to mercy killing, e.g., deliberately administering a lethal drug to a sufferer. Philosophers and, to some extent, physicians attempt to use the word with more exact meaning, even though there is little agreement about what that meaning is. They will distinguish between "voluntary and involuntary," "active and passive." Similarly, the terms "omission and commission" or "acting and withholding" are sometimes used. The definitions of all these terms are much debated. Even if they were clearly defined, merely using the right words would not make one decision ethical and another unethical. Rather than attempting to define the terms, we shall note those clinical situations where certain of these terms are likely to be used. Thus, the situations described in 1.5, in which a decision is taken to withdraw or withhold medical interventions of little utility, may be called "passive euthanasia." Some may call situations described in 2.5, in which patients refuse interventions that will keep them alive, "voluntary euthanasia." Others (ourselves included) wish to reserve voluntary euthanasia only for situations in which patients request that their life be ended by a lethal act. In situations in which the quality of a person's life is so compromised by pain and/or debilitation that a physician might be asked to kill the patient directly, the term "active euthanasia" might be used.

3.3.2 **"Active Euthanasia."** "Active euthanasia" is a phrase sometimes used to describe the situation in which someone (perhaps a physician) administers some lethal agent, e.g., a bolus of air, potassium chloride IV, excessive barbiturates, with the intention of causing the cessation of organic functions necessary to life.

CASE I. Mr. CARE is now suffering from advanced multiple sclerosis. He is bedridden and almost totally helpless. He asks his doctor to give him something to end his life, since he does not want to experience the progressive deterioration he knows he faces.

CASE II. Ms. T. O. is dying from widely disseminated cancer and is suffering intense and implacable pain. She begs her doctor "to put her to sleep forever."

3.3.3 **Moral Prohibitions.** Active intervention to cause or hasten death, whether done by a physician or by another, faces very strong moral prohibitions in our culture:

(a) Prohibition of the direct taking of human life, except in self-defense or in the defense of others, has been a central tenet of the Judeo-Christian tradition. It has been equally strong in the secular ethic.

(b) The ethics of medicine has traditionally emphasized the saving and preservation of life and has repudiated the direct taking of life. The Hippocratic Oath states, "I will not administer poison to anyone when asked to do so nor suggest such a course." The Judicial Council of the AMA states its interpretation of the professional ethics, "The intentional termination of the life of one human being by another—mercy killing—is contrary to that for which the medical profession stands and is contrary to the policy of the AMA." The weight of such statements must, of course, be assessed in view of the ethical arguments that support them. In our opinion and the opinion of most commentators, that weight is supported by valid arguments.

(c) The dedication of the medical profession to the welfare of patients and to the promotion of their health might be seriously undermined in the eyes of the public and of patients by the complicity of physicians in the death of the very ill.

(d) Even in particular cases, when effecting a swift death at the request of a suffering patient seems merciful and benevolent, the acceptance of the practice as ethical may bear the seeds of unacceptable social consequences. The "angel of mercy" can become the fanatic, bringing the "comfort" of death to some who do not so clearly request it, then to others who "would really be better off dead," finally to classes of "undesirable persons." The "euthanasia" program initiated in Germany in the early 1930s with the support of many benevolent physicians was first directed only to the incurably ill; it gradually expanded into genocide.

(e) Requests for swift death are often made in circumstances of extreme distress, which may be alleviated by skillful pain management and other positive interventions such as those developed by the Hospice movement. [3.4.]

COUNSEL. Physicians should take very seriously the ethical arguments against active euthanasia. These arguments appear to many commentators to add up to a decisive conclusion: Physicians have an ethical obligation to refrain from active euthanasia. Other commentators are not so absolute. They suggest that active euthanasia may be permissible in certain very restricted circumstances. Should any physician come to the conclusion in a particular case that he or she should accede to the plea of a sufferer who requests death, such a decision would be a sort of "conscientious objection" to the prevailing ethical and legal view. Conscientious objectors have a moral obligation to justify their act publicly and to accept the moral and legal consequences [2.10.1].

3.3.4 **"Death with Dignity."** The phrase "death with dignity" is sometimes heard in discussions of allowing to die and causing death. While appealing, the phrase is ambiguous and should not be allowed to carry weight in ethical deliberations without a precise definition of its meaning. If it is intended to mean that the expressed preferences of patients to refuse further medical intervention should be respected, "death with dignity" has important ethical significance: It is respect for the autonomy of the dying person. If it is intended to mean that dying persons should be spared the pain and inconvenience of repeated interventions of little utility, it also has ethical significance: It refers to the ethical obligation to shift from aggressive therapy to comforting care when therapy is futile. However, if it is intended to say that the suffering patient should be put "out of misery," it is ethically questionable and can be criticized by all of the arguments mentioned above. The phrase "death with dignity" should be reserved to describe the obligation to care for the dying sensitively, compassionately, and ethically.

3.3.5 **Legal Implications.** Deliberately causing the death of another constitutes a criminal act, as does cooperating in the causing of another's death. Thus, the physician who administers or provides a lethal agent is liable to a criminal charge of homicide or assisting suicide. Decisions to allow persons who are terminally ill to die, discussed in the previous chapters and sections, are also examples of "causing" the death of another. However, the clinical decision that further medical care would provide no therapeutic benefit other than to prolong organic life relieves the physician of the legal duty to continue to intervene with medical measures. This has long been considered an adequate defense against criminal and civil charges. A decision to kill the patient by using some lethal agent, even when death is imminent, does not rest on a clinical judgment about the futility of medical care. It is a decision that can be made by persons without medical skills, and the lethal agent can be a bullet, an electric shock, or rat poison. In such situations, anyone who kills another human being can be charged with a criminal offense: Physicians and laypersons alike must stand before the law. The "merciful" intent of the perpetrator is not a defense recognized by the law. However, in those few cases where physicians have been tried for "mercy killing," juries have acquitted them on grounds of insufficient evidence about the cause of death. Several laypersons who have been tried have been treated leniently on grounds of temporary insanity. Several efforts to enact statutes that would legalize mercy killing have been defeated.

3.4 PAIN RELIEF

In clinical situations a determination that the case is hopeless may lead to a decision to terminate life support. At the same time the patient may be conscious and in severe pain. Medication for pain relief is appropriate. Should it be provided up to the point where respiratory capacity is compromised, leading to death? This is a much debated question. It is clear that relief of pain is one of the major goals of medicine. It responds to the expressed preferences of the patient. It also improves the quality of life for the patient. On all these points, it is ethical. What is unclear is whether the side effect of analgesic medication, respiratory failure, should be considered as equivalent to active euthanasia.

3.4.1 **Skilled Use of Pain Medication.** This problem can often be avoided by intelligent and skilled use of pain medication. Unfortunately, intelligent and skilled use of these drugs is less common than could be desired. This lack, however, is increasingly recognized, and a literature is beginning to appear. Physicians should educate themselves and should seek consultation with persons expert in pharmacology and clinical pharmacy. Patients should not be kept on a regimen inadequate to control pain because of the ignorance of the physician or because of an ungrounded fear of addiction.

3.4.2 **Pain Relief and Maintenance of Compromised Functions.** On occasion, it is difficult to manage pain medication so that palliative effects and depressant effects are balanced. In such situations, should maintenance of adequate respiratory status take precedence over pain relief? Relief of pain and maintenance of compromised function are both goals of medicine. It can be plausibly argued that in the situation of the dying patient, the goal of maintenance of compromised function is itself related to the goal of prolonging life; prolonging life, in turn, is a goal that in this case has been properly abandoned. Thus, relief of pain becomes the primary goal to be sought during the remaining time of the patient's life.

3.4.3 **Double Effect.** The ethics of this problem are sometimes discussed in terms of "double effect." This is an ethical thesis that has been very much criticized. Still, its basic message has an appeal to clinicians. The argument stated here in outline is one that many ethicists still find persuasive.

Some actions have several effects that are inextricably linked. One of those effects is intended by the agent and is ethically permissible (e.g., relief of pain); the other is not intended by the agent and is ethically questionable (e.g., respiratory depression). Proponents of this argument state that the ethically permissible effect can be allowed, even if the ethically questionable one will inevitably follow, when the following conditions are present:

(a) The action itself is ethically good or at least indifferent, i.e., neither good nor evil in itself (in this case the action is the administration of a drug, a morally indifferent act).

(b) The agent must intend the good effects, not the evil effects, even though these are foreseen (in this case the intention is to relieve pain, not to kill the patient).

(c) The morally objectionable effect cannot be a means to the morally permissible one (in this case death is not the means to relief of pain).

In this argument the major practical problem for the clinician lies with the second condition (b), since often the intention of the physician is mixed: to relieve pain and to hasten death. If it can be said that the dosages administered are clinically rational, that is, no more drug is administered than is necessary for adequate pain relief, the intention to relieve pain seems primary and the action is ethical. If doses in excess of clinical necessity are given, the intention to hasten death seems primary. If this latter intention becomes primary, the action would be judged unethical. Roman Catholic medical ethics employs this argument to justify clinically appropriate pain medication for relief of pain, even if the unintended foreseen effect is the hastening of the patient's death. (EB: DOUBLE EFFECT.)

EXAMPLE. A 56-year-old woman suffers from carcinoma of the breast with lymphangitic spread to lungs and bony metastases. She requires increasing narcotic dosage for relief of pain. Her pulmonary function deteriorates so that her pO_2 is 45 and pCO_2 is 55 when she is pain-free [1.4–1.4.4].

COMMENT. Respiratory depression is the necessary side effect of appropriate dosages of morphine (i.e., sufficient to relieve pain). It is "unintended" in the sense that, if pain could be relieved by other means which would not have the effect, those means would be preferred.

3.4.4 **Diminution of Consciousness and Communication.** Attempts to achieve adequate relief of pain have another side effect, namely, the clouding of the patient's consciousness and the hindering of the patient's communication with family and friends. This double effect may be ethically troubling to the physician and to nurses. The dying patient will sometimes avidly desire communication and yet be in extreme pain. The patient may not be able to give directions about when, and to what extent, communication is preferred to pain. Those caring for the patient may have to make these decisions. In such situations no ethical principle will resolve the problem. Rather, sensitive attention to the patient's needs, together with skilled medical management, should lead as close as possible to the desired objective: maximum relief of pain with minimal diminution of consciousness and communication. Of course, if the patient is able to express preferences, these should be followed.

3.4.5 **Fear of Addiction.** It is very common that patients are not medicated adequately because of fear of addiction. This fear is irrational in the situation when death is imminent. Inadequate medication should be considered as unethical as overmedication.

3.4.6 **Physiological, Psychological, Social, and Spiritual Components.** Relief of pain is complex; it has physiological, psychological, social, and spiritual components. Attempts to deal with one factor alone in this complex network will often be futile. Thus, concentration on the physiological components of pain through pharmacological or surgical interventions, without equal attention to the psychological, social, and spiritual, may bring little relief. Even if relief is achieved in the physiological sense, other important ethical responsibilities may be left unfulfilled, e.g., aiding the patient to deal with his or her death and its effect on others. Physicians should make themselves aware of these components and seek assistance from those expert in dealing with them. The presence of religious counselors is often of immeasurable value to the patient, to the family, and to the physician.

3.5 SUICIDE

Suicide is the deliberate taking of one's own life. As an ethical problem, it should be discussed under patient preferences, Chapter 2. However, since the internist will often encounter the problem either at the end of the terminal illness of a patient, when life is of "poor quality," or in the emergency room, when preferences can only be inferred, it is discussed here.

There are significant ethical differences between suicide and the refusal of treatment:

(a) In refusal of care, a person does not take his own life; rather he does not permit another to help him survive. Persons who abhor the thought of suicide may say, "I do not want to kill myself. I only want to be allowed to die."

(b) In refusal of care, death is imminent from an irreversible disease; in suicide, although there may be irreversible disease, death is effected by some other self-inflicted lethal act. In refusing lifesaving care the patient does not set in motion the lethal cause; the fatal condition is itself the cause of death.

(c) Even though the result of suicide and refusal is the same, death, the moral setting differs completely in intention, circumstances, motives, and desires.

(d) The Roman Catholic Church, which adamantly condemns suicide, does permit its adherents to refuse care, even should death result, when treatment offers little hope and is burdensome, painful, or costly ("extraordinary") [2.6.1]. The California Natural Death Act, pioneer legislation in the matter of refusal of care, distinguishes between refusal of treatment and suicide, stating that any financial or legal penalities otherwise attendant on suicide do not apply to deaths resulting from refusal of treatment. (EB: SUICIDE.)

3.5.1 **Legal Considerations.** Suicide was long illegal in Anglo-American law. Suicides were punished by burial in unconsecrated ground; attempted suicides were considered felons. In the current century, laws against suicide were repealed in all states. The law now forbids assisting in a suicide. Physicians should refrain from assistance in suicide for the same reasons stated in 3.3.3 (active euthanasia).

3.5.2 **Treatment of Suspected Suicides.** Suspected suicides are frequently encountered in the emergency room. Even when the suspicion is supported by evidence, such as history and a suicide note, it has been customary to provide all means necessary for resuscitation and care, if there are solid medical grounds to expect recovery.

CASE. A 24-year-old woman is brought to the ER; she has deeply slashed her wrists and has overdosed. She has been brought several times before and is known to have a psychiatric history of depression. On her last admission she screamed that next time she should be allowed to die [1.3–1.3.3].

COUNSEL. The customary practice of disregarding the suicide wish in the emergency situation seems ethically appropriate, even though it seems to contravene the autonomy of the person.

(a) The ethical basis for suicide prevention is the well-known psychological thesis that the suicide attempt is very often a "cry for help" rather than an unambivalent decision to end one's life. Frequently the very fact that the attempted suicide arrives in the ER suggests the act was ambivalently motivated. Many suicides are made halfway. The suicide attempt may not be an act of autonomy but rather be an act resulting from impaired capacity due to some emotional conflict.

(b) Full circumstances surrounding the apparent suicide will rarely be known in the emergency setting. Thus, discrimination between genuine suicides and ungenuine suicides, as well as between suicides and acts of criminal battery, in the urgency of the emergency room would leave open wide possibilities for error, prejudice, and bias. The apparent suicide may not be a suicide at all.

3.5.3 **Ethical Obligation of the Physician.** Physicians have an ethical obligation to recognize the suicidal inclinations of patients whom they encounter in their practice and to make efforts to assist them personally or by referral to a psychiatric counselor.

BIBLIOGRAPHY

McCormick, R. The Quality of Life, the Sanctity of Life. *Hastings Center Report,* 1978, **8:**32.

McCormick, R. To Save or Let Die: The Dilemma of Modern Medicine. *JAMA,* 1974, **229:**172.

Fletcher, Jos. Indicators of Humanhood. *Hastings Center Report,* 1972, **2**(5):1. (In Shannon, 1976: 319.)*

Ramsey, P. *Ethics at the Edges of Life*. New Haven: Yale University Press, 1978, Ch. 4.

Shaw, A. Defining Quality of Life. *Hastings Center Report,* 1977, **7**(5):11.

3.2 *Quality of Life and Termination of Life Support*

Bayles, M. D. Euthanasia and Quality of Life. In Bayles, High, 1978: 128.

Brown, N. K., Thompson, D. J. Non-Treatment of Fever in Extended Care Facilities. *N Engl J Med,* 1979, **300:**1246.

Callahan, D. On Defining a Natural Death. *Hastings Center Report,* 1977, **7**(3):32.

Cassem, N. H. Controversies Surrounding the Hopelessly Ill Patients. *Linacre Q,* 1974, **42:**89.

Crane, D. Decisions to Treat Critically Ill Patients: A Comparison of Social Versus Medical Considerations. *Milbank Mem Q,* 1975, **53**(1):1.

Epstein, F. H. Responsibility of the Physician in the Preservation of Life. *Arch Intern Med,* 1979, **139:**919.

High, D. M. Quality of Life and the Care of the Dying Person. In Bayles, High, 1978: 85.

Paris, J. J. Withholding Life-supporting Treatment from the Mentally Incompetent. *Linacre Q,* 1978, **45:**237.

Suckiel, E. J. Death and Benefit in the Permanently Unconscious Patient. *J Med Phil,* 1978, **3:**38.

Skillman, J. J. Terminal Care in Patients with Chronic Lung Disease. *Arch Intern Med,* 1979, **139:**917.

3.2.1 *Legal Implications*

Annas, G. J. After Saikewicz: No-Fault Death. *Hastings Center Report,* 1978, **81**(3):16.

Annas, G. J. The Incompetent's Right to Die: The Case of Joseph Saikewicz. *Hastings Center Report,* 1978, **8**(1):21.

* Complete citations for abbreviated references appear at the end of the book under "General References."

Annas, G. J. Earle Spring and Quality of Life in the Courts. *Hastings Center Report,* 1980, **10**(4):9.

Annas, G. J. The Case of Brother Fox. *Hastings Center Report,* 1980, **10**(3):20.

Annas, G. J. In Re Quinlan: Legal Comfort for Doctors. *Hastings Center Report,* 1976, **6**(3):29.

Annas, G. J. Reconciling Quinlan and Saikewicz: Decision Making for the Terminally Ill Incompetent. *Am J Law Med,* 1979, **4**:367.

Baron, C. H. Assuring "Detached but Passionate" Investigation and Decision: The Role of Guardians ad Litem in Saikewicz-type Cases. *Am J Law Med,* 1978, **4**:111.

Beresford, H. R. The Quinlan Decision: Problems and Legislative Alternatives. *Arch Neurol,* 1976, **33**:371.

Buchanan, A. Medical Paternalism or Legal Imperialism: Not the Only Alternatives for Handling Saikewicz-type Cases. *Am J Law Med,* 1979, **5**:97.

Cantor, N. L. Quinlan, Privacy and the Handling of Dying Patients. *Rutgers Law Rev,* 1977, **30**:243.

Connery, J. R. The Quinlan Case. *Linacre Q,* 1976, **43**:25.

Hirsch, H. L., Donovan, R. E. The Right to Die: Medico-legal Implication of in Re Quinlan. *Rutgers Law Rev,* 1977, **30**:267.

Kennedy, I. M. The Karen Quinlan Case: Problems and Proposals. *J Med Ethics,* 1976, **2**:3.

Kittredge, F. I. After Quinlan. *J Legal Med,* 1976, **4**:28.

The Quinlan Decision: Five Commentaries. *Hastings Center Report,* 1976, **6**(1):8.

Relman, A. S. The Saikewicz Decision: A Medical Viewpoint. *Am J Law Med,* 1978, **4**:233.

Robinson, D. (ed.). *In the Matter of Karen Ann Quinlan.* Arlington, Va.: University Publications, 1975, 1976.

Robertson, J. A. Legal Norms and Procedures for Withholding Care from Incompetent Patients. In Abernethy, 1980:99.

Ryland, W. F., Baime, D. S. In Re Quinlan. *Rutgers-Camden Law J,* 1976, **8**:37.

3.3 *Euthanasia*

Alexander, L. Medical Science Under Dictatorship. *N Engl J Med,* 1949, **241**:39.

Beauchamp, Childress, 1979: Ch. 4.

Beauchamp, T. A Reply to Rachels on Active and Passive Euthanasia. In Beauchamp, T., Perlin, S. (eds.). *Ethical Issues in Death and Dying*. Englewood Cliffs, N.J. Prentice-Hall, 1978. (In Robinson, Pritchard, 1979: 182.)

Biomedical Ethics and the Shadow to Nazism. *Hastings Center Report,* 1976, **6**(4) (supplement).

Brandt, R. A Moral Principle About Killing. In Kohl, 1975: 106.

Cahill, L. S. A Natural Law Reconsideration of Euthanasia. *Linacre Q,* 1977, **44**:47.

Dyck, A. J. The Good Samaritan Ideal and Beneficent Euthanasia: Conflicting Views of Mercy. *Linacre Q,* 1975, **42**:176. (In Kohl, 1975: 117; in Horan, Mall, 1977: 348.)

Fletcher, Jos. The "Right" to Live and the "Right" to Die. In Kohl, 1975: 44.

Fletcher, Jos. Ethics and Euthanasia. In Horan, D. J., Mall, D. (eds.). *Death, Dying and Euthanasia.* Washington: University Publications of America, 1977, p. 293. (In Williams, 1974: 113.)

Fye, W. B. Active Euthanasia: An Historical Survey of Its Conceptual Origins and Introduction into Medical Thought. *Bull Hist Med,* 1978, **52**:492.

Husak, D. N. Killing, Letting Die and Euthanasia. *J Med Ethics,* 1979, **5**:200.

Kohl, M. (ed.). *Beneficent Euthanasia.* Buffalo: Prometheus Books, 1975.

Kohl, M. Voluntary Beneficent Euthanasia. In Kohl, 1975, 130.

Ladd, J. Positive and Negative Euthanasia. In Bayles, High, 1978, 105.

Meilaender, G. The Distinction Between Killing and Allowing to Die. *Theological Studies,* 1976, **37**:467.

Montague, P. The Morality of Active and Passive Euthanasia. *Ethics Sci Med,* 1978, **5**(1):39.

O'Rourke, K. D. Active and Passive Euthanasia: The Ethical Distinctions. *Hosp Prog,* 1976, **57**(11):68.

Rachels, J. Active and Passive Euthanasia: *N Engl J Med,* 1975, **292**:78. (In Robeson, Pritchard, 1979: 153.)

Ramsey, P. The Indignity of Death with Dignity. *Hastings Center Report,* 1974, **2**(2):47. (In Horan, Mall, 1977: 305.)

Rosner, F. The Jewish Attitude Toward Euthanasia. *NY State J Med,* Sept. 1967, 2499.

Russell, B. On the Presumption Against Taking Life. *J Med Phil,* 1979, **4**:244.

Sherwin, B. L. Jewish Views of Euthanasia. In Kohl, 1975: 3.

Steinbock, B. The Intentional Termination of Life. *Ethics Sci Med,* 1979, **6**:59.

Trammel, R. L. The Presumption Against Taking Life. *J Med Phil,* 1978, **3**:53.

Walton, D. N. Active and Passive Euthanasia. *Ethics,* 1976, **86**:343.

Zaner, R. (ed.). Appraisals (articles on death and dying). *J Med Phil,* 1979, **4**.

3.3.5 *Legal Implications*

Baughman, W. H. Euthanasia: Criminal Tort. *Notre Dame Lawyer,* 1973, **48:**1202.
Euthanasia (special issue). *Baylor Law Rev,* 1975, **27**.
Kamisar, Y. Some Nonreligious Views Against Proposed "Mercy Killing" Legislation. *Minnesota Law Rev,* 1958, **42:**969. (In Horan, Mall, 1977: 406)
Louisell, D. W. Euthanasia and Biathanasia: On Dying and Killing. *Catholic University Law Rev,* 1973, **22:**723. (In Horan, Mall, 1977: 383.)

3.4 *Pain Relief*

Ashley, O'Rourke. 1978: Ch. 13–14.
Churchill, L. R. Interpretations of Dying: Ethical Implications for Patient Care. *Ethics Sci Med,* 1979, **6:**211.
Dunphy, J. E. On Caring for the Patient with Cancer. *N Engl J Med,* 1976, **295:**313.
Garfield , C. A. *Psychosocial Care of the Dying Patient.* New York: McGraw-Hill, 1978.
Gorovitz, S. Dealing with Dying. In Bayles, High, 1978: 29.
Hackett, T. P. Psychological Assistance for the Dying Patient and His Family. *Ann Rev Med,* 1976, **27:**371.
Hudson, R. P. Death, Dying and the Zealous Phase. *Ann Intern Med,* 1978, **88:**696. In Bayle, High, 1978: 65.
Krant, M. J. The Hospice Movement. *N Engl J Med,* 1978, **299:**546.
Lamerton, R. *Care of the Dying.* London: The Priory Press, 1973.
Lewis, G. The Place of Pain in Human Existence. *J Med Ethics,* 1978, **4:**122.
Mount, B. M. et al. The Management of Intractable Pain in Patients with Advanced Malignant Disease. *J Urol,* 1978, **120:**720.
Noyes, R., Travis, T. A. The Care of Terminally Ill Patients. *Arch Intern Med,* 1973, **132:**607.
Saunders, C. Hospice Care. *Am J Med,* 1978, **65:**726.
Smith, H. L. The Minister as Consultant to the Health Team. *J Religion and Health,* 1975, **14:**7.
Twycross, R. G. The Assessment of Pain in Advanced Cancer. *J Med Ethics,* 1978, **4:**112.
Twycross, R. G. The Use of Analgesia in Terminal Illness. *J Med Ethics,* 1975, **1:**10.

Vanderpool, H. Y. The Ethics of Terminal Care. *JAMA,* 1978, **239:**850.
Wilson, J. M. Communicating with the Dying. *J Med Ethics,* 1975, **1:**18.

3.4.3 *Double Effect*

Beauchamp, Childress. 1979: Ch. 4.
Ashley, O'Rourke. 1978: 194.
Boyle, J. M. Toward Understanding the Principle of Double Effect. *Ethics,* 1980, **90:**527.
Foote, P. The Problem of Abortion and the Doctrine of Double Effect. *Oxford Review,* 1967, **5:**5. (In Gorovitz, 1976: 267.)
Graber, G. Some Questions About Double Effect. *Ethics Sci Med,* 1979, **6:**65.
McCormick, R. A. *Ambiguity in Moral Choice.* Milwaukee: Marquette University Press, 1973.
Ramsey, P., McCormick, A. (eds.). *Doing Evil to Achieve Good: Moral Choice in Conflict Situation.* Chicago: Loyola University Press, 1978.

3.5 *Suicide*

Beauchamp, Childress. 1979: 85–94.
Grisez, G. Suicide and Euthanasia. In Horan, Mall, 1977: 742.
Hook, S. The Ethics of Suicide. In Kohl, 1975: 57.
Lebacqz, K., Englehardt, H. T. Suicide. In Horan, Mall, 1977: 669.
Perlin, S. (ed.). *Handbook for the Study of Suicide.* New York: Oxford University Press, 1975.
Ruben, H. L. Managing Suicidal Behavior. *JAMA,* 1979, **241:**282.

4

EXTERNAL FACTORS

4.0 This chapter discusses "external factors" that may be considered when ethical decisions about patients must be made. These external factors include (a) the role of the patient's family, (b) the costs of medical care, (c) the allocation of medical care, (d) research values, (e) teaching values, and (f) the safety and well-being of society. The question raised by all these factors is whether, and to what extent, burdens and benefits accruing to persons other than the patient should ever be relevant or decisive in clinical decisions regarding the patient.

All of the ethical principles previously discussed in this book underlie the problems of this chapter. However, the principle of utilitarianism, i.e., those actions are ethically right which contribute to the greater good of the greater number, is particularly relevant. This principle may, in some of its interpretations, appear to conflict directly with the duty of a physician to benefit and not to harm the individual patient who is being cared for. Also, ethical doctrines of justice, requiring fair distribution of social benefits, may propose policies that appear incompatible with the physician's duty to individual patients. It is the purpose of this final chapter to state some of those situations where clinical benefits and social benefits might appear to dictate different courses of action. It is our opinion that the principle of duty to the patient's welfare should prevail in almost all circumstances. The circumstances in which we favor benefit to others than the patient are stated. If our counsel seems at times somewhat uncertain, it is because some of these situations do pose genuine dilemmas. (EB: ETHICS; UTILITARIANISM; HEALTH POLICY; JUSTICE; SOCIAL MEDICINE.)

4.1 FACTORS INFLUENCING PATIENT–PHYSICIAN RELATIONSHIP

Medicine has traditionally concentrated on the medical needs of individual persons as these persons have sought medical care. The care and cure of individuals were its objectives. Medical care, however, does not take place within the isolation of a one-on-one encounter between patient and physician. Family, friends, institutional arrangements, social structures, cultural values, economic conditions—all these influence the patient–physician relationship. It has also long been recognized that many factors external to the person are important for the understanding and management of his or her illness and for the promotion of health. However, in the physician's efforts to assist a patient, the interests of persons other than the patient have played a very limited role. The exercise of clinical discretion requires a precise knowledge of what that role should be.

4.1.1 **Definition of External Factor.** For the purposes of this chapter, "external factor" refers to any result of a clinical decision that can constitute a benefit or burden to some party other than the patient about whom the decision is made. Although almost every decision will have some external effects of this sort, the question is whether the physician should explicitly consider these effects and allow them to influence or determine the clinical decision. Is it ethically permissible to weigh the patient's interests against the interests of other persons or society?

That such weighing does take place is obvious. In some instances it leads to clearly unethical practices; in others it is more ethically ambiguous and sometimes has the appearance of virtue.

EXAMPLE I. Medicare patients coming to a particular clinic with a complaint of back pain are given a much more extensive battery of diagnostic tests, some of which entail risk, than non-Medicare patients. Reimbursements for these unnecessary and risky tests accrue to the financial benefit of the medical staff of the clinic.

EXAMPLE II. A 72-year-old man who is senile suffers from severe emphysema. He is being cared for, with great difficulty, by his 74-year-old wife, who is becoming increasingly distraught. Still, she insists she does not want him to go into a nursing home. When the patient develops pneumonia, it occurs to the physician that "his death would certainly be a great relief to his wife."

COMMENT. In the first example an external factor, profit, rather than the patient's need, dictates diagnostic decisions. This is clearly an illegal and unethical practice: The ethical strictures on physicians have traditionally prohibited unnecessary procedures for profit. In the second example an external factor, the burdens borne by the elderly, devoted wife, will certainly elicit the sympathy of the conscientious physician. However, it is not entirely clear whether this consideration regarding the wife should influence the physician's decision about the patient's care. [Cf. 4.2.6–4.2.7.]

EXAMPLE III. The current interest in the costs of medical care and the allocation of resources sometimes leads physicians to ask, "Is it not costing society too much to continue this treatment for this patient? We have better use for our resources. We should stop now." Comments such as these require that we ask whether an external factor, the cost of an individual patient's care and the burden these costs lay upon society, should dictate clinical management. [Cf. 4.4.]

The question then should be: Is it ever ethical to make a clinical decision contrary to the interests of the patient, or one that does not promote the patient's interests, in order to foster the interests of some other person or institution? If it is sometimes ethical to do so, what considerations justify such a decision?

4.1.2 **Differentiation Between Clinical Discretion and Health Policy.** It is important to note that this chapter is still about the *clinical discretion* of physicians in managing individual patients. It is *not* about health policy. This chapter's comments are applicable only to the clinical situation. Quite a different framework of thought must be devised to deal with questions of health policy and the ethical issues raised by policy proposals. Even though clinical decisions and policy decisions are related in intricate ways, policy decisions are made in different ways, for different purposes, and in a different atmosphere from clinical decisions. Thus, when a policymaker asks "whether better use for resources exists than (say) neonatal intensive care or CAT scanners," the answer depends upon many facts and considerations not available to the clinician. Further, the policymaker is accountable to the public in a much more visible and definitive way than is the clinician. The physician is accountable to the individual patient and not to the public.

EXAMPLE. Mrs. COPE, the noncompliant diabetic [2.8], is now hospitalized for treatment of severe ketoacidosis. Ulcerations on her legs, incurred during a recent alcoholic episode, are not healing. She develops acute renal failure. The Renal Fellow says, somewhat in jest, "We really ought to reduce the burden on the End-Stage Renal Disease Program. Somehow dialysis has to be rationed. We ought to start here."

COMMENT. The jocular remark of the Fellow would, if taken seriously, substitute a concern about the national policy governing the use of an expensive resource for the interests of the patient who is his responsibility. If the same remark, without reference to any individual patient, was made by the Assistant Secretary for Health, DHHS, it would express a legitimate policy concern and would be answered, after extensive study, by devising a program that would be both cost-effective and fair.

The legitimacy of the DHHS officer's remark, in contrast to that of the Renal Fellow, rests on at least three reasons:

(a) The former is a public statement, susceptible to public analysis and criticism; the latter is made in private, providing no opportunity for public scrutiny.

(b) The former would be pursued by determining standards and procedures and specific criteria for inclusion and exclusion of recipients of care; the latter appears to issue from emotion and prejudice, outside any context of standards, procedures, and criteria.

(c) The former represents the role and task of a DHHS officer —"it's his job to deal with such problems"; the latter in no way represents the role and task of physicians (unless they are also public officials) in our society—"it's not his business."

4.1.3 **Creation of Ethical Problems by Institutions and Policies.** It is also important to note that many of the ethical problems raised by clinical decisions about particular patients are caused by social policies and the structure of institutions. For a variety of reasons, such as limited fiscal resources or political pressures, social and institutional policies will favor some groups at the expense of others. *Example:* Patients with end-stage renal disease are the object of a public program specially designed for them; patients with hemophilia do not enjoy such a program. The result may be that the hemophilia patient has more difficulty obtaining adequate treatment and institutions have more difficulty providing them adequate care.

This may lead to clinical decisions about such patients that are forced by the circumstances of social policy and financial resources. Individual physicians may be able to do little about these circumstances. Thus, the physician may be faced with undesirable options for ethical choice. Although we are vividly aware that inequitable, inefficient, or inadequate social policies do create situations where all ethical options are less than ideal, this chapter does not discuss the reform of social policy. This is a problem that must be taken up elsewhere. This chapter deals only with the clinical decisions themselves.

4.1.4 **Relevance of External Factors.** It is tempting but simplistic to say that external factors should never be allowed to influence a decision about a patient: Only the patient's welfare, not the welfare of others, should be the clinician's objective. This is tempting because it reflects the traditional Hippocratic ethic of patient benefit. It is simplistic because holding so absolutely to a principle, in this case as in others, creates situations that appear to almost every rational observer as unethical.

> EXAMPLE. A physician in 1904 stood by silently while a young man whom he knew to have syphilis married without telling his fiancée his condition. The physician wrote: "A single word would save her from this terrible fate, yet the physician is fettered hand and foot by his cast iron code . . . he cannot lift a finger or utter a word to prevent this catastrophe" (Bok, 1978, p. 147).

The point of this example is not to ask whether or not the physician was right in maintaining confidentiality. It is cited merely to show that observing an ethical principle can create an objectively evil situation. The question, then, is whether the principle should be applied in a particular situation. In answering that, we must consider such factors as the harm caused by its application and the burdens or harms (or benefits and profits) that come to other parties. These, then, are relevant considerations in the deliberations. The difficult problem is whether these considerations should ever be *decisive*.

> EXAMPLE. Should the burden imposed on the elderly devoted wife [4.1.1(II)] be the decisive consideration in deciding not to treat her husband's pneumonia? Should the high cost of the End-State Renal Disease Program be the decisive factor in excluding Mrs. COPE from dialysis [4.1.2; 4.5]?

4.1.5 **Decisiveness of External Factors.** The most serious question is whether external factors should ever be decisive in clinical decisions that are ethically problematic.

> CASE I. The 29-year-old retarded man described in 3.1.1(IV) develops acute lymphoblastic leukemia. His parents are unwilling to continue to bear the burden of his care. They refuse permission for treatment of leukemia. Should the external factor, i.e., the burden imposed upon the parents, be the decisive consideration in deciding not to treat?

As a general principle, we propose that external factors should not be decisive over consideration of (1) medical indications, (2) patient preference, (3) quality of life. However, external factors may move toward greater decisiveness in clinical decisions when all of the following conditions are met:

(1) The achievement of significant goals of medical intervention is doubtful [1.1.3].

(2) The preferences of the patient are not and cannot be known [2.2.5].

(3) The quality of the patient's life approaches the threshold considered minimal [3.1.5].

In the example of the retarded person with acute lymphoblastic leukemia, the burden imposed upon parents is a relevant and important consideration. However, it should not be decisive because (1) significant medical goals can be achieved and (2) the quality of the patient's life, while poor, is not close to the minimal threshold.

> CASE II. Mrs. C. Z., a 35-year-old woman, has been through several courses of chemotherapy for Hodgkins disease to no avail. Her tumor is now staged at IVB. She has decided to discontinue chemotherapy and accept only palliative care. While in the hospital for treatment of severe edema of the neck and cellulitis, she chokes on soup and, before an airway can be opened, suffers five minutes of anoxia. Several weeks later she is on a respirator and has been described by the neurologists as being in a persistent vegetative state. Her husband insists she be kept alive. The costs of her care now approach $12,600. Should the respirator be turned off?

COMMENT. In this case, two external factors, the wishes of the husband and the costs of care, deserve consideration. The considerations directly relevant to the patient lead to the following conclusions: (a) The indications for medical intervention bear only on the minimal goal of treatment, namely, preservation of organic life; no other goals are attainable. (b) The preferences of the patient are not known and cannot be ascertained. (c) The quality of her life is at, or below, the threshold considered minimal. In such a situation, the wishes of her husband to continue, while *important,* are not decisive. The costs of care and the allocation of resources are decisive. Each of these factors will now be discussed in particular.

4.1.6 **External Review of External Factors.** In the usual course of the practice of medicine, important decisions are, and should be, made by the patient and the physician together. Outside parties have no right to partake in those decisions unless invited to do so by the principal parties. However, when external factors become relevant to a particular clinical decision under the circumstances mentioned above, a strong case can be made for the more prominent role of external parties. The presence of external factors raises the issue of conflict of interest, since someone other than the patient will bear burdens or enjoy benefits resulting from the decision. One traditional means of preventing conflict of interest from leading to results harmful to one of the principals is review by persons who do not have an interest in the outcome. Thus, when discussing various external factors, we suggest some sort of external review is often advisable. The involvement of third parties in clinical decisions is not customary in medicine (although the consultant sometimes plays a role). However, in an era when external factors have assumed growing influence on the patient–physician relationship, we believe external review, when appropriate, can provide balance, dispassionate advice, and protection to all parties. Common forms of external review are the appointment of guardians or conservators, the judicial proceeding, committees (such as those now existing for human experimentation), and formal processes of administrative review. In many cases this review will be advisory, and the primary physician will retain the authority to make the clinical decision; in other cases the external reviewer will be empowered to make the decision, as in guardianships [cf. 1.8; 2.2; 4.2.1].

4.2 ROLE OF THE FAMILY

Many patients have close family who are intimately involved in the illness and in the medical care of their relative. Often family members take on an important role as decisionmakers for the patient who may be severely compromised physically, mentally, or emotionally by illness. What is the *legal* standing of family members in crucial decisions? What is the *moral* standing of family?

4.2.1 **Legal Authority of Family.** Family members and next of kin have *no legal authority* to make crucial decisions on behalf of *adult* patients unable to make decisions on their own behalf, unless that authority is specifically given by the act of a judge granting guardianship powers (or in several states, by a statute).* Parents or guardians do have legal authority by statute to make decisions for minors, with some limitations [2.7.3].

Physicians *must not assume* they have a legal duty to obtain permission of next of kin to perform medical acts for an incapacitated patient. It is, of course, always advisable to consult with next of kin. In certain situations, it is prudent to recommend that a legal guardianship be obtained by a family member for the specific purpose of making decisions regarding medical care. This should usually be done when there is question of a major intervention, such as elective surgery or embarking on a course of chemotherapy for an incapacitated patient.

In the case of Mrs. C. Z. mentioned above [4.1.5], the husband has no legal authority to determine whether treatment continue or cease. Physicians have no legal duty to act in accord with his wishes. He may seek and be granted such authority after petitioning a judge, who may require a hearing. Other parties, such as her parents or her physician, might also petition for legal guardianship.

4.2.2 **Moral Authority of the Family.** In American culture, the moral authority is significant, although it is perhaps less dominant than in other cultures. Physicians should pay close attention to family wishes in situations where the patient is unable to make decisions. These wishes are ethically *important* primarily because they may reflect the personal preferences of the patient who is, at present, unable to express them. Family may be the best source of information about their relative's preferences, judgments of quality life, and so forth. If patient preferences are one of the most ethically decisive factors in treatment decisions, any evidence about them when the patient cannot express them is important.

CASE. An 83-year-old woman suffers extensive chest and pelvic trauma when hit by a car. She is on a respirator in the

* Maine, Idaho, North Carolina (1979).

ICU. She is somewhat confused and disoriented. However, she continues to write notes saying, "I want to die" and "Leave me alone." Her two sons and one daughter arrive from a distant city. They state their mother was a very independent lady until her accident. She is intelligent and well informed. She has said to them many times, "I don't want to be dependent. I don't want to deteriorate. I don't want to be like my sister" (who was severely debilitated by a stroke for seven years before her death) [1.3–1.3.3].

COMMENT. The testimony of the sons and daughter is important evidence of their mother's preferences. There is no reason to suspect it is false or to suspect them of ulterior motives. If they had merely said, "She should be allowed to die; she'd be better off dead than deteriorating," they might have been expressing *their* preferences rather than *hers*. The expression by family of the patient's preferences is clearly relevant and may be decisive. The expression of *their own* preferences is less important ethically and may not even be relevant.

4.2.3 **Conflict of Interest.** Conflict of interest or other sorts of biases in the expressions of family about their ill relatives may be suspected. If the suspicion is well grounded, their statements about their relatives should not be considered relevant to decisions about their care.

CASE I. A 76-year-old man is found in his boardinghouse room comatose, hypothermic, emaciated, and with gangrene of toes on both feet. After being taken to the hospital, he is found to be in renal failure. Social workers contact his family, a son and a daughter. The former operates a successful business in a neighboring state; the latter is a prominent local socialite. On arriving at the hospital, they insist that "everything be done to keep their father alive." The daughter expresses surprise that he is so ill since, "while I don't see him very often, I had always told him to get in touch if he needed me" [1.4–1.4.4].

CASE II. The same as Case I, with these modifications: The patient, despite living in poverty and isolation, is known to have a considerable fortune. His son and daughter tell you,

"You must let him die in peace. His last years have been so miserable."

COMMENT. In both versions of the case there is reason to suspect the son and daughter are not acting in the best interest of their father. In the first version, guilt over neglect may supply strong self-interested motives; in the second the prospect of inheritance may do so. This does not mean a decision to treat in version I or not to treat in version II would be wrong; it simply means that such a decision should not be based on the wishes of next of kin. Rather, the questions of direct patient welfare, raised in Chapters 2 and 3, are much more important and, in most cases, should be decisive.

COUNSEL. Family wishes should be considered *important* in clinical decisions about patients unable to express their preferences when (1) there is no reason to suspect bias or conflict of interest, and (2) relatives show evidence of close and continuing concern for the patient.

4.2.4 **Best Interests of the Patient.** Decisions made by others about the patient should always be in the patient's best interest. Obviously, what constitutes "best interest" may be controversial. Is continued painful treatment with little hope of cure, but with the effect of prolonging life, in the patient's best interest? Is death ever in a person's "best interest"? Determination of best interest, for practical purposes of clinical decisions, should look to the following:

(a) It can be presumed that attainment of the goals of medical intervention would be in the interest of the patient. If significant goals are unlikely to be attained, treatment may not be in the patient's interest [1.1.3].

(b) If only the minimal goal, maintenance of organic life, can be attained, it can be reasonably argued that continued treatment is not in the patient's interest (since it can be argued that no truly personal life remains, thus, no personal interests can be promoted) [3.1.5].

(c) Since persons define their own interests, is there any direct or indirect evidence about how this patient defined interests? If no such evidence exists and if significant medical goals are not being attained, as described in (a), it can be concluded that treatment is not in the patient's interest [2.0–2.1.7].

(d) If there is evidence, e.g., a relative's report or a document, and that evidence shows a preference for treatment (even a treatment which others might consider useless), those preferences should be respected unless heavy costs and burdens are imposed on others.

Thus, relatives may suggest, and physicians accept, certain treatment decisions that meet the above conditions; these decisions could be said to be in the patient's interest and, as such, reflect the ethical principle of respect for the autonomy of the patient.

4.2.5 **Ignoring the Patient.** Health professionals sometimes attend to family wishes while neglecting the actual patient.

EXAMPLE. An elderly person is brought to a clinic for medical care. The doctor does not acknowledge the presence of the elderly person. He addresses all questions to her daughter. The elderly person does not appear to be mentally incapacitated but sits quietly while her daughter and the doctor converse. Elderly patients are often treated as if they were incompetent or are infantilized by health professionals. This is a serious failure to respect that patient as a person.

4.2.6 **Relief of Others as a Consideration in Patient Care.** Even when family do not express any wishes, the physician may be aware of the burdens imposed on a family or spouse by the impaired life of their relative. Relief of others is often an *important* consideration leading to change in regimen or arrangements for care. Should it ever be *decisive* in deciding not to treat?

CASE I. A 67-year-old man, who has had a brilliant artistic career, suffers from advanced senile dementia. His devoted family is extremely distressed. His children believe their mother is being precipitated into a breakdown. At present the man is in the hospital with pneumonia. The family halfheartedly tells you to do your best for him [1.4–1.4.4].

CASE II. The same as Case I, except there are no children and the husband has been cared for during the last two years by his wife, who herself suffers from severe arthritis and is now exhausted. Since they live in the country, transfer to a nursing home would mean separation.

COMMENT. In Case I, the decision to treat the patient's pneumonia should consider the full range of therapeutic possibilities for this patient (a CARE patient). The goals of restoration of health and maintenance of compromised function will not be achieved. In addition, this episode of pneumonia is likely to be followed by another. On the other hand, he is still relatively young and healthy in all respects except for his somewhat early senility. His life, while of low quality, cannot be considered of minimal quality. Finally, the family situation suggests alternative arrangements for the care of their father can be made and the mother relieved of the burden. In our opinion, the external factors are not sufficiently weighty to justify a decision not to treat this man's pneumonia.

In Case II, separation of this couple may have serious consequences for both. If both together could be domiciled in a nursing home, the problem would be resolved. If this were impossible, the prospect of separation from her living spouse may be more difficult for this woman than his death. This question should be explored with her. Should she agree, it is our opinion that it is ethically permissible not to treat the patient's pneumonia. His own irreversible illness offers only a limited achievement of medical goals. The quality of his life is progressively deteriorating. His preferences are not known. In addition, the serious burden that his care imposes on this ill, exhausted, yet devoted wife bring these external factors, in our opinion, to a decisive point.

4.2.7 **Relief of Others as a Decisive Consideration.** Even if ethically permissible (and some will argue it is not permissible at all), the decision in 4.2.6 (II) is troubling. In this case the medical indications, looked at in isolation, call for treatment. The patient's preferences are not known. Quality of life, while poor, is not minimal. A role greater than usual is given to the decision of the spouse. In such a situation, where, despite appearances, the possibility for conflict of interest is great, some external review might be advisable. This could be done informally, by requesting the advice of a disinterested but sympathetic person, such as a clergyman, by requesting Ethics Committee review, or, more formally, by the appointment of a conservator. [Cf. 4.1.6.]

4.2.8 **Organ Transplantation.** The transplantation of tissue from one living person to another involves a medical intervention that puts one person, the donor, at risk (without compensating medical benefit) in order to benefit another, the recipient. This is an unusual situation in medical ethics, which traditionally has not allowed the physician to "do harm" without also benefiting the actual patient. Although some early commentators raised questions about the ethical propriety of being a donor and accepting an organ, today this practice is widely considered ethically permissible and praiseworthy. However, it cannot be so easily shown that any person has an ethical *obligation* to donate an organ. Donation should be a free and generous gift. Nevertheless, strong social and psychological pressures bear on the potential donor in many situations. The internist may occasionally be involved as a consultant and adviser to a potential donor.

CASE. Ms. J. P., a 28-year-old divorced woman, comes to her primary care physician for advice. Her 25-year-old brother, an only sibling, has been found to be in renal failure. He and her parents, as well as the nephrologist, have urged her to be tested for suitability as a donor. She is extremely anxious and says that while she feels guilty, she does not want to be a donor.

COMMENT. It is common in ethics to distinguish between duties and altruism or "acts of supererogation." A person is said to have a duty when another person has a strict right to the performance of some action by the first party. An act of supererogation is done not out of duty but out of generosity; no one has a corresponding right. It is important to maintain this distinction in organ transplantation. The suggestion that an afflicted person has a "right" to the organs of another specific living person has obvious and troubling consequences. In a recent judicial decision, the court implicitly relied upon this ethical distinction in refusing to order a person to "donate" bone marrow to a relative dying of leukemia. Even such a relatively risk-free intervention, with the possibility of significant benefits for the recipient, should be "an act of supererogation."

COUNSEL. The primary care practitioner in the case above is the physician for the woman, not for her brother. "He owes the patient his primary allegiance" (AMA Judicial Council, Organ Transplantation Guidelines). He may explain to her the risks of being a donor as accurately as possible. He should explore her motivations and fears, as well as the details of her relationship with her family. He might even comment on the desirability, from a medical viewpoint, of the transplantation. He cannot, however, maintain a purely neutral stance since, as her physician, he has an obligation to be her advocate. If she finally decides not to undergo the tests, the physician should support her and be her ally in dealing with family and the specialist. (EB: ORGAN TRANSPLANTATION.)

4.3 CONFIDENTIALITY

There is a duty incumbent on the physician to maintain in confidence all information learned from or about the patient. This obligation is justified by the right of privacy, by the expectation of the patient, and by the social advantages of the practice of confidentiality. Questions about confidentiality arise when maintaining it might have a harmful effect on another or breaching it might benefit others. In some situations protection of the public is the central issue. In many cases, however, the person who will benefit or be protected by having the information will be a family member. The exceptions to confidentiality for protection of the public are discussed in 4.8. Confidentiality in the family situation is represented by the following cases. (EB: CONFIDENTIALITY; PRIVACY.)

CASE I. A 46-year-old man is diagnosed as being in imminent danger of myocardial infarction. He commands the physician not to inform his wife.

CASE II. A 32-year-old man is diagnosed as suffering from Huntington's chorea. He commands the physician not to inform his wife, whom the physician knows is eager to have children.

CASE III. A 43-year-old man is treated for gonorrhea ten days after returning from a business trip. He insists that his wife not be informed.

COMMENT. In general, the personal assurance of confidentiality (a sort of implicit promise) and the social advantage of maintaining confidentiality require strong justification for any exception. In principle, the *well-founded expectation* of *serious harm to another specific party* (not others in general) is the most justifiable ethical reason to breach confidentiality. Thus, Case I, in which the wife may benefit by knowing of the husband's illness, does not exemplify a strong justification. His illness does not pose an imminent danger for her. If unusual circumstances existed, e.g., the couple was about to depart on a cross-country automobile trip during which he would be the driver, justification for revealing the condition is stronger. The imminent, serious, and likely harm to the wife (from gonorrhea infection) or to future children (from genetic disease) creates stronger justification. Obviously, in any such situation, if the same effect (i.e., protection of another from harm) can be attained without breaching confidentiality, every effort should be made to do so. Such efforts should themselves be ethically proper, avoiding deception and coercion. *Example:* The physician calls the wife of the man in Case III and tells her to come in for a shot, because "something is going around." This stratagem is not only inept but also a deception, which in the long run may cause more harm than it avoids.

Note: Cases of exceptions to confidentiality are sometimes the most excruciating of ethical dilemmas. The strong obligation to the patient is directly countered by a strong obligation to another innocent party in danger of serious harm. When a true dilemma is posed, a conscientious decision in either direction is ethically permissible: no consideration is decisive for one over the other.

Other questions arise about confidentiality when protection of the public is an issue [cf. 4.8].

4.4 COSTS OF CARE

Costs are incurred whenever medical care is provided. Costs are incurred by patients or their families who pay out of pocket; by insurers who recover in premiums paid by the insured; by local, state, and federal governments, which recover them in taxes paid by the public.

Almost 90 percent of Americans have some form of health insurance, although coverage is often quite incomplete. Since 1965 the substantial share of medical bills incurred by persons over 65 has been paid by a federal program, Medicare. Medicaid is a joint federal and state program to pay for the care of the poor. Qualifications for this program and coverage differ from state to state.

4.4.1 **Costs to Individuals.** Despite the existence of private insurance and public programs, individuals still bear a considerable portion of the cost of medical care. In some instances these costs can be excessive and even ruinous. Individuals may not seek, or may refuse, needed care to avoid these costs.

> CASE. A 63-year-old man, recently retired from his own small business, is diagnosed as suffering from acute nonlymphoblastic leukemia. He has never had adequate health insurance and has only $10,000 in savings. He is not old enough to be eligible for Medicare. He decides to spend his savings on a world cruise with his wife rather than enter chemotherapy. Being a Catholic, he consults his priest, who affirms that his decision is in conformity with the Catholic teaching that medical care, even lifesaving, which in the judgment of the person is too costly can be considered extraordinary and thus not morally obligatory [2.6.1]. The gentleman and his wife enjoy a three-month tour, and two months after returning he becomes seriously ill and dies.

COMMENT. In this case, the costs of care fall directly upon the patient. He exercises his personal autonomy by preferring the world cruise to therapy that might prolong his life. His own preference is sustained by the teaching of his church. The cost of care, in this case, is decisive in the patient's ethical judgment to refuse treatment. In this sense, then, the statement that the cost of care may justify not providing that care is certainly acceptable: The patient who bears the burden makes the decision. The patient's physician may consider such a decision foolish or shortsighted but should respect the decision as an act of the patient's autonomy [cf. 2.5].

4.4.2 **Costs Incurred by Family.** Costs for the care of a relative may be excessive and compromise the attainment of other legitimate goals of the family. They may feel that other needs and obligations, such as education of children, supersede the duty to provide treatment that is of little or no benefit.

CASE. Parents of four children, aged seven to 18 years, earn a moderate income by both working. They have modest savings and no investments other than home and car. The husband's mother, aged 60, has had two successive mastectomies, followed by chemotherapy for metastases. Her hospital bill is in excess of $30,000. She is now confined to a nursing home and is mentally incapacitated. She develops colonic and rectal cancer. Her son is asked whether surgery should be performed.

COMMENT. This lady's son may determine that the costs of continued treatment for his mother would be ruinous for his own family, particularly jeopardizing the education of his children. Indications for treatment are questionable but not absent; the patient's preferences are unexpressed; the quality of her life is poor but possibly can be improved with treatment. However, there are real and urgent obligations to specific others. In our opinion, this fact, added to the above considerations, does justify the son's recommendation not to proceed with treatment. It must be hoped that arrangements could be made to avoid this tragic situation. Physicians have a moral obligation to assist in making alternate arrangements.

4.4.3 **Costs to Society.** It is widely recognized that the costs of medical care constitute a major problem for the American economy and society. (EB: HEALTH CARE; THEORIES OF JUSTICE.)

EXAMPLE. The End-Stage Renal Disease Program, instituted in 1972 to relieve patients of the heavy costs of dialysis and

> transplantation, was originally estimated to cost $250 million by 1976. By 1980 it was costing $1 billion for the care of 50,000 patients. These patients are less than 0.2 per cent of Medicare eligible patients, but they receive more than 4 per cent of Medicare outlays.

Cost of care, in terms of the federal budget or as a percentage of the gross national product, is a problem of public policy. It can be dealt with only on the basis of policy-relevant data and policy analysis. Thus it is necessary to know how these costs are generated, what accounts for their increase, and what sort of economic effects flow from current or alternative policies. As a policy problem, it is a matter for policy makers, not clinicians. It is not relevant to clinical decisions except in two specific ways:

(a) Cost containment [4.4.4]
(b) Rationing [4.5]

4.4.4 **Cost Containment.** Efforts to contain costs may be applied at various levels. At the policy level a federal program may provide greater incentives for less costly care than for other forms; at the clinical level, an effort might be made to provide care more efficiently.

> EXAMPLES. In the End-Stage Renal Disease Program, incentives favor facility dialysis, the more expensive form of care, over home dialysis. This could, presumably, be rectified. Similarly, a hospital may include in its formulary only generic drugs when available and equivalent to brand-name drugs. Cost-containment efforts can reach the level of clinical decision when an effort is made to reduce the number of diagnostic tests or the number and type of drugs prescribed by house officers. The presumption behind all these efforts, essential to a judgment about their ethical nature, is that the alternatives chosen as less costly are, in fact, equivalent in safety and efficacy to the more costly ones. This is a factual determination, about which arguments can often arise. However, if good reasons can be alleged in favor of equivalence, no ethical problem is generated by cost-containment efforts. The claim that such efforts are unethical may rest more on the physician's lack of confidence and knowledge than on any genuine danger

to patients. Rationing of medical care raises other and quite genuine ethical questions.

4.5 ALLOCATION OF SCARCE RESOURCES

Rationing can have the broad meaning of allocation of any limited resource by any allocation mechanism, such as the market. As such, rationing is the pervasive activity of economic life. Rationing may have the more specific meaning of allocating some limited resource in terms of a plan that states criteria and priorities. Gasoline and food rationing in wartime is of this more specific type.

4.5.1 **Rationing of Medical Care.** Medical care has always been a scarce resource. The number of physicians, the location of their practice, the ability of persons to pay, the different perceptions of medical need—these factors and many others lead to certain allocations of medical care resources. However, in recent years the specific question whether medical resources should be allocated by a plan stating priorities and preferences has been raised. This is a troubling question for physicians who have adhered to the traditional medical ethic of "rendering to each [patient] a full measure of service and devotion" (AMA Principles of Medical Ethics). In one sense, no physician renders a "full measure" to any one patient, since physicians have many patients, all of whom must be served. Thus physicians have traditionally rationed their time and efforts. Still, the idea of a plan for rationing medical services is troubling to physicians.

EXAMPLE. One way of limiting the excessive costs of the End-Stage Renal Disease Program would be to set up criteria that would identify acceptable patients. These criteria might look to the age of the patients, the presence of complicating disease, the coping abilities of the patients, the presence of supporting "networks" of family, and so on. Patients who met these criteria would be admitted for dialysis; others would not.

COMMENT. The setting of criteria would be done not by the clinicians directly responsible for the patient but by program administrators. Use of criteria, however, would be in the hands of the clinicians. Even though an impersonal "other" would rule out the person seeking care as ineligible, the clinician would have to inform the person. Presumably the physician would make exceptions, legally or otherwise. Thus, even policy determinations reach the level of clinical decisions. Questions of "triage," of competing claims, and of selection will face the clinician in some form (EB: RATIONING OF MEDICAL TREATMENT.)

4.5.2 **Triage.** Medical care has long been provided in accord with a plan in one specific situation, battlefield medicine. Since the Napoleonic Wars, military doctors have established priority rules for the treatment of casualties ("triage" is the French word for selection). In recent years triage rules have been refined and applied to other disasters, such as earthquakes and hurricanes. The rules of triage and its rationale are stated in a handbook of military surgery:

> Priority is to be given to (1) the slightly injured who can be quickly returned to service, (2) the more seriously injured who demand immediate resuscitation or surgery, (3) the "hopelessly wounded" or the dead on arrival . . . . The military surgeon must expend his energies in the treatment of only those whose survival seems likely, in line with the objective of military medicine, which has been defined as "doing the greatest good for the greatest number" in the proper time and place. [Emergency War Surgery (Washington, D.C.: U.S. Government Printing Office, 1958), pp. 168, 33.]

EXAMPLE. During World War II, triage decision was made at the policy level to provide penicillin, in extremely short supply, first to soldiers with venereal disease rather than to the wounded, since the former could be more quickly returned to battle readiness (and were also infectious).

4.5.3 **Criteria for Triage.** The citation of the Utilitarian Principle [4.0] in a handbook of military surgery, "the greatest good for the greatest number," makes clear the ethical principle of triage: to return to service those who are needed for the victory, a common good for the army and the nation. Similarly, disaster triage provides priority to persons such as firemen, public safety officers, and medical personnel in order for them to be returned to rescue work. Present disaster and serious danger to the society justify triage rules. This notion is lost in the more casual use of triage, e.g., the "triage nurse" in the ER or the application of triage rules to the allocation of intensive care beds apart from emergency situations. Lacking the element of present disaster and the destruction of the fabric of social order, rules that subordinate the needs of individuals to the needs of society are not easily justified in medical ethics.

COUNSEL. When treatment or nontreatment decisions must be made on a triage basis, the following conditions should be observed:

(a) There should be an immediate and severe danger to the fabric of society, such that the threat to the society's survival is clear and present.

(b) The selection of certain persons on the basis of their position or skills should be based on the judgment that they will quickly return to their posts.

4.5.4 **Competing Claims to Care.** Situations arise when it can be asked whether the claims of one patient for care override the claims of another. Personnel, time, equipment, beds, and other factors are insufficient to accommodate both. In addition the common-good justification for triage is not present; this is a competition between two rival claimants. In passing, it might be noted that such situations are often avoided by "finding a way" by use of stratagems that nurses, in particular, seem particularly ingenious in devising.

CASE I. Mrs. C. Z., the patient described in 4.1.5, has suffered prolonged anoxia. In this version she is not in persistent vegetative state but has been in deep coma for seven days. She is sustained on a respirator in the Intensive Care Unit of a small community hospital in a rural area. The victim of an automobile accident is brought to the hospital with a crushed chest, apparent pneumothorax, and broken bones in the extremities. This patient requires a respirator immediately. Mrs. C. Z., of the six patients on the six respirators in the unit, has the poorest prognosis. Should she be removed in favor of the accident victim?

COMMENT. The medical prognosis of Mrs. C. Z. is very dismal. Prolonged anoxia has left her severely damaged. She may soon die or slip into persistent vegetative state, although there is also the unlikely possibility she may emerge from coma. In addition, her death from Hodgkins disease is certain and probably will occur soon. Her preferences about her care and her life are unknown. Given these considerations, the immediate and serious need of an identifiable other person becomes an important consideration. When that person is in imminent danger of death, the extrinsic factor of scarcity of resources becomes decisive in the decision regarding Mrs. C. Z. It is ethically permissible to remove her from the respirator.

CASE II. Mrs. M. T., a 52-year-old woman, has had GI bypass surgery for excessive obesity. Following the surgery she has had innumerable complications requiring twelve further operations and three years of almost constant hospitalization. The cost of her medical care has now reached $200,000. She is in need of hyperalimentation but refuses to learn how to care for herself. She has become very dependent on the staff and the institution. She is extremely demanding, critical, and querulous. She also eats surreptitiously. Daily wound care is required for fistulae. [1.4–1.4.4.]

COMMENT. Mrs. M. T.'s care is a considerable drain on the time and energy of all who care for her. It is the perception of the staff that other patients are suffering from diminished attention. The achievement of medical goals is limited to palliative care. Mrs. M. T.'s preferences are ambiguous: She wants care but will not take responsibility for her health. The quality of her life is poor but does not approach minimal. In this case the competing others are not single identifiable persons in urgent need, but any patient who happens to pass through that service. They suffer from a compromised level of care due to the overextension of the staff but are not in danger of death or serious harm.

COUNSEL. It is ethically permissible to discharge Mrs. M. T. There is no certainty she will do herself harm by eating, even though this can be suspected. She may be stimulated to begin to take care of herself. The staff has no obligation to provide domiciliary care in order to protect Mrs. M. T. against herself and her irresponsibility. She may harm herself if discharged; the staff will not harm her. On the other hand, Mrs. M. T. is doing harm to others with rightful claims on the resources of the unit.

CASE III. Patient R. A., the drug addict described in 2.8.2, is in need of a second prosthetic heart valve. Several physicians are strongly opposed to providing a second prosthesis. These physicians offer three reasons: (1) Surgery is futile, since the patient will become reinfected; (2) the patient does not care enough about himself to follow a regimen or to abstain from drugs; (3) it is a poor use of societal resources.

COMMENT. The first and second considerations are discussed in 2.8.2. The third consideration raises new ethical issues. (1) What are the criteria for differentiating good from poor uses of societal resources? Statement of such criteria leads to the problems noted in 3.2.4–3.2.5. (2) There is no guarantee that whatever is "saved" by refusing this patient will be used in any better manner. (3) The resources are, of course, not being "absorbed" by the patient; they are flowing to the hospital, to the physicians and surgeons, to nurses, and so on. Complaints about wasting resources should not be made without recognizing that the "wasted" resources support, in large part, the medical care system.

COUNSEL. The most acceptable ethical justification for refusing to provide a second prosthesis is the medical indication that the risks of surgery and its attendant mortality exceed the risks of managing the patient with medical therapy. Thus, if medically indicated, the surgery should be offered. The ethical obligation to provide surgical assistance is, however, diminished to the extent that the rights of other patients are directly compromised, as explained in *Comments* to Cases I and II, 4.5.4.

4.5.5 **Admission to Programs with Limited Resources.** Medical care is so organized that certain procedures and therapeutic programs are available only at a few locales or from a few specialists. More persons may need this sort of care than can be accommodated. How should the resources be allocated? All commentators on the ethics of this problem agree that resources should be allocated in a fair manner: What constitutes fairness?

EXAMPLE. When chronic hemodialysis became available in the late 1960s, the very limited resources required some rationing device. A local committee was established to screen all applicants who had been judged acceptable on medical grounds. The committee was forced to rely on "social worth" criteria, that is, personal and social characteristics that merited the treatment. This technique proved unworkable and was much criticized for bias and prejudice.

COMMENT. Extensive ethical discussion of this issue seems to have reached consensus on the unacceptability of the social worth criteria as a principle of fair distribution. Some commentators have favored "queuing" (first come, first served) although they note that these systems favor the better informed and better connected, who can hurry to the queue. Many favor a lottery, whereby all participate in a drawing of random numbers. This system, however, is faulted because all the pool of needy persons does not exist at any one time. In the most extensive program requiring allocation of scarce resources, the renal transplantation program, selection is now facilitated by the international computerized system for tissue typing. This introduces a major objective consideration, which obviates the biases of social worth and also reduces the uneasiness of having life and death depend purely on "the luck of the draw."

COUNSEL. The dangers of bias and prejudice inherent in a social worth system advise its rejection as a rationing device. It seems most fair to establish certain very basic objective criteria —e.g., medical condition, potential for benefit, and age—and within a pool of those who meet these criteria to select randomly. It may also be useful to establish a "due process" system, which could make exceptions to the randomization. If this is done, the criteria for exception should be based on the triage model, 4.5.3.

4.6 RESEARCH VALUES

Many patients are treated under formal research protocols. Care of cancer patients, in particular, may take place within a program for evaluation of chemotherapy. Other patients also present an opportunity to obtain information useful for the treatment of future patients. Research values accrue to persons other than the subject of research, namely, to future patients, to the professional doing the research, and to society in general. Even when the subject personally benefits—for example, goes into remission as the result of treatment with an experimental drug—these others are also beneficiaries. Should research values ever be relevant to, important for, or decisive in decisions about care of a particular patient? (EB: HUMAN EXPERIMENTATION; INFORMED CONSENT IN HUMAN RESEARCH.)

4.6.1 **Definition of Clinical Research.** Clinical research is defined as any maneuver or intervention that has as its primary objective the development of generalizable knowledge (National Commission for the Protection of Human Subjects of Biomedical and Behavioral Research).

4.6.2 **Regulation of Clinical Research.** Clinical research is governed by guidelines stated in several ethical codes (Nuremburg, Helsinki, AMA). Regulations promulgated by the Department of Health and Human Services are mandatory for all federally funded research and, in many institutions, for all research. They require:

(1) Review of proposed research by an Institutional Review Board made up of experts—biomedical scientists as well as some "outside" persons. This IRB must evaluate the risks and benefits of the research procedures and recommend approval or disapproval to the funding agency.

(2) Informed consent by any competent participant and permission by guardians for incompetent persons (with special review

and protection procedures in specific cases). Many of the ethical problems regarding research must be resolved in the course of review, e.g., an appropriate risk-benefit ratio, the details of appropriate disclosure, the suitability of compensation.

4.6.3 **Clinical Research vs. Innovative Treatment.** It is difficult to distinguish research from innovative treatment. In innovative treatment, for example, a physician may choose to employ a drug, approved for other purposes, for a condition in which it has never been used. The clinician may do so primarily as a last resort in the care of a particular patient and without the intention of developing generalizable knowledge, even though the clinician may be able to draw some conclusions in retrospect. In research the intent to develop generalizable knowledge is primary and instigates the development of a research plan and the use of methodologies useful in the gathering, analysis, and validation of information. Innovative treatment is not, as such, governed by the codes and regulations that govern research. However, it should be governed by the same spirit. The advice of knowledgeable colleagues should be sought, a risk-benefit ratio as accurate as possible should be worked out, and the consent of the patient to be the subject of a yet untried treatment should be obtained. In addition, innovative treatment should be designed as closely as possible to research, so that the social benefit of valid knowledge can be obtained. Finally, in doubtful cases, clinicians should seek the advice of the IRB about the advisability of innovative treatment.

4.6.4 **Ethical Problems in Clinical Research.** All clinician-researchers should honor the ethics of clinical research by abiding by the requirements of informed consent of subjects and review of protocols by competent bodies. However, in clinical situations ethical problems may still arise. It might be asked whether a particular patient, who is in general an appropriate candidate for an approved protocol, should be approached because the risk-benefit equation is questionable in this patient's case.

This problem might arise in situations in which a new drug, believed to be of potential benefit from preliminary animal and human investigations, is to be compared in a formal clinical trial against a placebo.

> EXAMPLE I. When the polio vaccine first became available, it was tested in large surveys against a placebo. Many clinicians believed in the efficacy of the vaccine and were concerned that some preventable poliomyelitis—including paralysis and death—would occur in the control subjects who did not receive the actual vaccine.

COMMENT. Randomized clinical trials are a relatively recent development. They are essential to the development of effective and safe medical (and surgical) therapies. Many ethical problems exist in such randomized trials. In double-blind trials, neither the doctor nor the patient knows whether the patient is receiving a drug or a placebo. Some physicians find this situation clinically and ethically unacceptable. Some physicians are concerned that their patients may be randomized to an inferior therapy. However, a properly designed controlled trial would be one in which a true null hypothesis exists so that neither of the proposed therapies could be regarded as definitely better than the other. In the early polio vaccine trials, it is worthwhile to recall, a large number of subjects who received the actual polio vaccination may also have been injected with another live virus, the long-term effects of which are not yet entirely clear.

Also, prejudice about efficacy can cause considerable harm. The problem of retrolental fibroplasia in the early days of neonatology is a tragic example: "A simple example of clinical delusions about therapeutic preferences occurred when the administration of oxygen to premature babies was suspected of causing the epidemic of retrolental fibroplasia that took place about 20 to 25 years ago. At first, when the oxygen was regarded as desirable, a controlled trial was opposed because the 'control' babies would be denied a beneficial treatment. Later, when the oxygen was regarded as hazardous, a controlled trial was opposed because the treated babies would be needlessly exposed to danger" (Feinstein, 1977).

It can be asked whether patients should be continued on protocol, or new patients entered, when a clinician-researcher believes the majority of patients whom he has treated seem to benefit from one experimental drug rather than the standard treatment (presuming the clinician is not "blinded" to the randomization or, if "blinded," is suspicious).

> EXAMPLE II. The University Group Diabetes Program (UGDP) was a multicenter study in which patients with diabetes were randomized to several treatment programs, one of which involved the use of oral hypoglycemic agents. In one of the medical centers involved in the study the senior investigator concluded that there appeared to be a higher mortality among patients on oral hypoglycemics than among patients being treated with insulin. His center then broke the randomization and withdrew from the multicenter trial on the grounds that it was ethically wrong to treat patients in a manner (i.e., with oral hypoglycemics) that appeared to increase their risk of heart attacks and death.

COMMENT. In this instance the senior investigator at one of the many centers involved in the project weighed the possibly detrimental effect on research of breaking the randomized trial and withdrawing his institution from the clinical trial against his allegiance to his patients' welfare. In this calculation, the investigator considered his patients' welfare to be paramount. This required that he discontinue the research and treat all the patients with insulin. Without commenting on the scientific merits of the investigator's analysis of the research, we believe his actions were ethically commendable in view of his understanding of the situation. The patients' interests were placed above those of scientific research, and this is how medicine—both clinical and investigative medicine—should be practiced. However, the accuracy of clinical impressions in large trials can be questioned. Also, the import of statistical methodology, e.g., setting levels of significance, must be carefully examined.

COUNSEL. It is advisable to establish an independent monitoring group to which data can be made available without breaking the blinding. Various methods, such as sequential analysis, are often appropriate statistically and ethically and can reveal trends.

4.7 TEACHING VALUES

Many patients receive care in institutions where clinical teaching is done. Their disease and its diagnosis and treatment provide an opportunity for students in the health sciences to learn the skills necessary for their profession. Often, actual treatment will be provided by a student. It is possible that some clinical decisions are made with a view to these teaching values and that such decisions may conflict with the patient's interests and/or wishes. (EB: MEDICAL EDUCATION.)

CASE I. A 52-year-old obese woman required a lumbar puncture. The procedure was supervised by a second-year resident attended by four medical students. It was performed on a shaky bed in a four-bed ward without draping. The resident left the room after giving instructions to the students and watching one of them make several unsuccessful attempts to insert the needle in the spinal canal. "You've got to start somewhere," the resident remarked.

COMMENT. There is no ethical *problem* in this case; it is an ethical outrage. No consideration was shown to the patient's feelings, supervision was inadequate, easily arranged accommodations were not made. Students are often offended by being placed in such situations. As low persons in the medical school hierarchy, students may feel an ethical conflict and not know how, and to whom, to express their feelings.

Although the case described is an outrageous example of an ethical insult, we must be aware that relatively inexperienced students perform many procedures in teaching hospitals, including blood drawing, I.V. insertions, lumbar punctures, paracenteses, thoracenteses, and occasional endotracheal intubations. Students often remark (in private) about their feelings concerning these procedures. They are eager to learn these skills and believe they must master these techniques in order to function effectively as physicians. Still, they are not sure how to approach the patient and how much disclosure is appropriate for the patient's informed consent, particularly for relatively innocuous albeit discomforting procedures, such as venipuncture.

CASE II. A 74-year-old man with chronic obstructive pulmonary disease is admitted in mild respiratory failure and with diffuse bronchospasm. His respiratory condition probably does not require emergency intubation. The therapeutic options include medical management and observation in an effort to avoid or postpone intubation. After considering the situation, the chief resident orders early intubation, and one of his reasons for this choice is to allow an inexperienced intern to practice intubating a patient.

COMMENT. Procedures involving any risk should be performed only for diagnostic or therapeutic purposes. Risky procedures should not be done exclusively or even partially for their teaching value. Thus, in Case II, the intern's need for additional practice in intubation should not be a relevant consideration in the chief resident's clinical judgment. If the procedure is harmless, such as palpation or auscultation, or involves only minor inconvenience, such as asking a patient with ataxic gait to get up from his chair and walk across the room, or minor discomfort, as extension and flexion of an arthritic limb, patients may be requested to allow the procedure. Harmless procedures may also be done on patients who are mentally incapacitated.

4.7.1 Consent. Patients should give their consent to be teaching subjects. Persons who enter teaching hospitals usually sign a general consent to that effect. Many patients, particularly those who are seriously ill at the time of admission or who for other reasons are unable to comprehend the meaning of the teaching hospital consent form, have probably not given adequate informed consent to be used as teaching subjects. They should be asked specifically about each episode of teaching. The demonstration procedure should be explained to the patient; the fact that the procedure will be done by a student and that it is for teaching rather than for their care (or in addition to their care) should be made clear. The request should be made politely and a refusal accepted graciously. Patients are amazingly generous in consenting to participate in the education of medical students in teaching hospitals. On the occasion of the history taking and physical diagnosis course, many patients provide their histories to five or more students without complaint. In the light of these observations, it is particularly important that, when the occasional patient refuses to participate in one or another teaching exercise, the student and the faculty respect that patient's wishes absolutely and not threaten or intimidate the patient in any way. Medical students and physicians must remember that *individual* patients are not obligated to participate in the training of society's future physicians. They almost invariably are eager to do so, and physicians should be sensitive to their enormous debt to patients for the patients' unquestioning generosity.

Many patients enjoy being asked to be teaching subjects. Medical students often pay them more attention than their regular physician, particularly in teaching settings. This is a patient benefit. However, it should not of itself be presumed as the justification for using patients for teaching purposes.

> CASE III. A chief of cardiology at a major teaching hospital is concerned over the high rate at which coronary artery bypass grafts become occluded soon after surgery. The cardiologist suspects the problem results from the way the venous graft was removed from the thigh vein, the way it was handled, and then the way the graft was sutured into the coronary circulation. The cardiologist knew many of these procedures were done by surgery residents and fellows who were supervised by the senior attending cardiac surgeon. The cardiologist is perplexed. On the one hand, his own research and training program in academic cardiology depends on having available an active group of cardiac surgeons. On the other hand, the cardiologist feels that, in view of the poor surgical results at his institution, he could not recommend his own patients to the surgical service for their coronary artery surgery. Tension between the needs of patient care and those of teaching are quite apparent.

COMMENT. For the time being the cardiologist should not send his patients to a surgical group with poor results and perhaps poor techniques. This surgical training program would improve only by being denied cases from medical cardiology. The problems seem to be technical in nature, and technical errors are often the easiest to correct in a medical setting. The best medical teaching is conducted in clinical settings that provide excellent medical care.

4.8 SOCIAL CONSIDERATIONS

On certain occasions benefits and harms to the society other than those discussed above appear to result from treatment decisions. The classic example is the protection of a population from the threat of disease by quarantine or by immunization.

Quarantine of carriers of infection is a treatment decision for the benefit of persons other than the patient: The patient's liberty is restricted in an effort to protect the public. This is also the case with mandatory immunization. Similarly, the reporting of infectious diseases to the health department is required by law in most jurisdictions. This also is intended to warn and to provide preventive or therapeutic measures to persons other than the patient. At the same time the confidentiality due the patient is compromised. Finally, dangers of other sorts, such as the violent threats of a patient to do bodily harm to others, may recommend forms of treatment, from involuntary detention to use of tranquilizing or antipsychotic drugs. What are the conditions that justify any treatment decision which appears to be more beneficial for others than for the patient? Is it ever justified to make a decision clearly not for the patient's benefit but for the wellbeing of others? (EB: PUBLIC HEALTH; SOCIAL MEDICINE.)

CASE I. The student in 1.3 has meningococcal rather than pneumococcal meningitis. He refuses therapy and wishes to return to the dorm.

CASE II. A 28-year-old man who has been under your care for severe peptic ulcer impresses you as somewhat bizarre in attitude and behavior. You suspect that he suffers from a psychotic disorder and ask him whether he is seeing a psychiatrist. He calmly responds that he was once under treatment for schizophrenia but has been well for years. Then, in the course of an office visit, he casually tells you he would like to see the mayor dead and was thinking of assassinating him. Should you report your patient to the police?

CASE III. A 27-year-old nurse in a dialysis unit is hepatitis

B antigen positive. She is reluctant to inform her social contacts and resists any restriction of her professional activities. She approaches a private practitioner for advice. If she is adamant, should the practitioner take steps to ensure that her social contacts are informed of her condition? Should the practitioner take steps to see that her professional activities are restricted?

COMMENT. In Case I, meningococcal meningitis is an infectious disease. Infectivity is high and thus the return of the student to the dormitory puts fellow students at high risk of a serious disease. Protection of specific others from a serious harm justifies the decision to detain the student and to treat. In Case II the danger to others is less clear. This patient is obviously in need of psychiatric treatment and should be persuaded to seek it. The threat, as is often the case, may be empty. Several of the conditions that would justify breach of confidentiality are present: An identifiable person is threatened, and serious harm could be done. The absent condition is assuredness about the likelihood of the patient's taking action. The consequences to the patient of being reported to the police might be significant. The consequences of reporting "suspicious persons" on the basis of suspicions aroused in medical care encounters might also be socially undesirable.

In Case III the infectivity of the nurse is low; the possibilities for contact are extensive and difficult to limit. She is capable of arranging her social contacts so as to avoid infecting others. In terms of her personal life and social behavior, the matter should be left to her own responsibility. In terms of her professional life, she has a direct obligation to protect her patients from harm. If she refuses to do this by reporting herself and by restricting her activities voluntarily, the physician has a duty to report her.

COUNSEL. The ethical obligation to protect others, even at the expense of interfering with the patient's liberty and privacy, is strongest in Case I: There is a genuine threat of serious harm to particular, identifiable persons. In Case II we do not consider the likelihood of harm sufficiently great to justify a breach of confidentiality, although in that situation, many circumstances may heighten assurance that the patient is very likely to act out his fantasies. In Case III, the more remote risk, the responsibility of the person for her own behavior and the practical impossibility of protecting everyone with whom she deals do not add up to an obligation to protect others, except the patient population with whom this person deals as a health professional.

4.8.1 **Legal Implications.** Most jurisdictions have statutes requiring the physician to report cases of certain sorts, such as venereal disease, gunshot and knife wounds, and child abuse. These statutes should be obeyed when the physician has practical certainty that the reportable fact is present. Exceptions should not be lightly made. (Many physicians will fail to report child abuse or venereal disease, particularly when the parents or patients are ''respectable''; this failure is reprehensible.) In some places reporting practices have fallen into disuse or follow-up procedures by health departments are nonexistent or casual. Where a report would be useless, the obligation of confidentiality rules. Most jurisdictions also have statutes allowing physicians to detain persons and to treat them when such persons are dangerous to themselves or others. These statutes usually set out specific conditions and limits. Physicians should acquaint themselves with the precise provisions of these statutes in the jurisdictions in which they practice. [Cf. 2.7.2.]

In one precedent-setting case, Tarasoff v. Regents (1976), a student informed his psychotherapist that he intended to kill a young woman. This was not communicated to the woman, who was subsequently murdered. The California Supreme Court ruled that the psychiatrist and the psychologist had a positive duty to take reasonable steps to protect third parties from harm. This *may* include warning the victim or notifying the police. The serious danger of violence to an identifiable person was a consideration which, in the opinion of the court, overrode the obligation to preserve confidential information obtained in the course of psychiatric therapy. In the court's opinion, existence of such a duty would not deter persons from seeking help from psychotherapists. Thus, the revelation of confidences would not be socially detrimental. It is unclear how this decision would apply to an internist or a general practitioner who obtains similar information in the course of providing general care. However, an internist should seek consultation from persons expert both in mental health and in the law. Every effort should be made to obtain psychiatric help for the patient. If the internist judges the threat to be real and likely to be carried out, the matter should be reported to authorities. (EB: CONFIDENTIALITY.)

4.8.2 **Conflict of Interest for the Physician.** The occupational physician, the military physician, and the prison or police physician may encounter conflicts of interest. As physicians they are obliged to serve those who come to them as patients; as employees they have some obligations to their employers. Ethical problems may arise, particularly about confidentiality and disclosure.

CASE I. The dialysis nurse described in 4.8 is examined by the hospital's Employee Health Service physician. This examination is required by hospital regulations. When the physician tells the nurse she is hepatitis B antigen positive, she insists he not report her to the director of the dialysis unit.

COMMENT. The physician in this case has accepted responsibilities to the institution as well as responsibilities to particular patients. This dual relationship should be clear to the patient in this situation. The physician should report this patient. The dual relationship may not be clear in many situations where workers approach company physicians. It is imperative that the dual relationship be made clear whenever it is relevant and that its implications be spelled out for the patient-employee.

CASE II. A worker in an industry using kepone visits the company physician about a persistent cough. The physician does a cursory physical and prescribes a cough medicine. It is company policy not to investigate symptoms of this sort too aggressively until they become demonstrably more serious. It is also policy not to suggest to worker-patients the potential for lung disease or to make employee health records available to them.

COMMENT. The company policy is manifestly unethical since it causes persons who may be benefited by early diagnosis and treatment to be deprived of it through remediable ignorance. The physician who accepts such a policy clearly acts unethically, since duties to patients are disregarded without the patient's being made aware of the physician's dual role.

4.8.3 **Code of Ethics.** The American Society for Occupational Medicine endorses a Code of Ethics that states the obligations of physicians who are in a dual relationship. In part, the Code states:

> 1. accord highest priority to the health and safety of the individual in the workplace;
> 4. actively oppose and strive to correct unethical conduct in relation to occupational health services;
> 5. avoid allowing their medical judgment to be influenced by any conflict of interest;
> 7. treat as confidential whatever is learned about individuals served, releasing information only when required by law or by over-riding public health considerations, or to other physicians at the request of the individual according to traditional medical ethical practice; and should recognize that employers are entitled to counsel about the medical fitness of individuals in relation to work, but are not entitled to diagnoses or details of a specific nature.
> 9. communicate understandably to those they serve any significant observations about their health, recommending further study, counsel or treatment when indicated. [Code of Ethical Conduct for Physicians Providing Occupational Medical Services. From *Journal of Occupational Medicine,* Volume 18, No. 8, August 1976.]

This code does not resolve the ethical problems of physicians who, in attempting to follow it, jeopardize their position. It is our belief that such ethical problems should always be resolved in favor of patients; we recognize that doing so may lead to disadvantages and perhaps suffering on the part of the physician. Physicians accepting positions with dual responsibilities should be certain that their employers will allow them to abide by the ethical code.

4.8.4 **Torture and Punishment by Physicians.** It should go without saying that physicians employed in prisons and by police should not participate in interrogation and punishment of suspects and convicts. Under no circumstances should they participate in torture. They should not participate in civil executions, except to declare death, which they alone can do under the law in most jurisdictions. In these activities there is no patient benefit. (EB: PRISONERS.)

4.8.5 **Strikes by Physicians.** In recent years physicians have organized to withhold medical services for a period of time in order to win concessions for themselves or for patients. *Examples:* All anaesthesiologists in a particular state agree not to assist at any elective surgery in order to protest excessive malpractice insurance premiums; all physicians of a province agree not to provide anything but emergency services in order to protest the level of reimbursement for patient care provided in the health insurance plan of the country; the house officers of a city hospital refuse to provide anything but emergency care in order to protest the inadequate facilities, working conditions, and staffing of the institution.

The form of withholding services is crucial. Thus, reasons of self-interest are much less weighty than reasons of correcting genuine deficiencies in patient care. Withholding only services not urgently needed is more justifiable than withholding all services (a distinction that may be difficult in practice). Nevertheless, the fact that the withholding of service penalizes particularly vulnerable persons, namely patients and potential patients, makes concerted withholding of services ethically dubious even when justifications are strong. In general, physicians have, as a group, considerable social authority and political influence in our society. They have many means of redressing inequities short of withholding their services.

4.9 OTHER EXTERNAL FACTORS

Many external factors other than those discussed above affect clinical decisions. Physicians, like all persons, have to allocate their time, attend to personal and family affairs, and earn an income. They work within certain administrative structures and within certain relationships with peers. They are affected by public policies, such as the institution of federal programs like Medicare or the rates of reimbursement for certain procedures. In addition, their habitual or occasional emotional and psychological states influence their decisions. While it is not possible here to analyze these factors, their presence and influence on decision making should be noted and, in particular situations, carefully scrutinized.

In general, external factors like those mentioned above should not be important considerations in ethical decisions about patients. On occasion they may become important.

> EXAMPLE. An inadequate level of Medicare reimbursement never justifies inadequate care to patients; it may, however, be an important consideration in deciding whether to limit the number of such patients one can serve.

On very unusual occasions, one of these factors may become decisive. *Example*. Family ties would not usually be a relevant consideration in deciding how to allocate one's time among patients, but a physician would be ethically justified, in an accident, in attending his own children before other injured persons.

4.10 SOCIAL RESPONSIBILITIES

This book has discussed only the ethical problems encountered in clinical decisions about individual patients. However, physicians also have social responsibilities as citizens. Some of these responsibilities arise from the knowledge and skills proper to the medical profession and from the expectations the public has about the profession's function in society. Physicians, as individuals and as organized groups, should take positions on activities and policies that have implications for the health of the society. Traditionally the profession exercised leadership in efforts to protect communities from quackery, from communicable disease, and from contaminated food and water. Today professional leadership should be exerted in such areas as health education about personal behavior; the use of tobacco, alcohol, and drugs; housing and nutrition; environmental pollution; highway safety; occupational safety; and domestic and military nuclear policy. Physicians also exercise considerable authority over the ways in which medical care is organized. The profession bears a corporate responsibility to assure that the provision of care is not dominated by self-interest rather than the health needs of the public. Finally, the profession continues to enjoy broad autonomy in determining standards of care and over the admission, education, and discipline of physicians. It thus bears the responsibility for maintaining high standards, effective programs of physician education at every level, and a fair but efficacious disciplinary system for the protection of the public. (EB: SOCIAL MEDICINE; POVERTY AND HEALTH; PUBLIC HEALTH; WARFARE; RACISM AND HEALTH; ALCOHOL, USE OF; DRUG USE; ENVIRONMENTAL ETHICS; FOOD POLICY; POPULATION ETHICS.)

BIBLIOGRAPHY

4.0 Jonsen, A. R., Jameton, A. R. The Social Responsibility of Physicians. *J Phil Med,* 1977, **2**:376.

4.2 cf. bibliography at 2.7–2.7.3.

4.2.8 *Organ Transplantation*

Beauchamp, Childress, 228–33.*

Calland, C. H. Iatrogenic Problems in End Stage Renal Failure. *N Engl J Med,* 1972, **287**:334.

Feinberg, J. Supererogation and Rules. *Ethics,* 1961, **71**:276.

Fellner, C., Schwartz, S. Altruism in Dispute. *N Engl J Med,* 1971, **284**:582.

Fellner, C. Organ Donation: For Whose Sake? *Ann Intern Med,* 1973, **79**:590.

Fox, R. C., Swazey, J. P. *Courage to Fail.* Chicago: University of Chicago Press, 1974.

Freund, P. Organ Transplants: Ethical and Legal Problems. *Proceedings Am Phil Soc,* 1971, **115**: 276. (In Reiser, Dyck, Curran, 1977: 171; in Gorovitz, 1976: 535.)

Katz, J., Capron, A. M. *Catastrophic Diseases: Who Decides What?* New York: Russell Sage, 1975

Kelly, G. The Morality of Mutilation: Towards a Revision of the Treatise. *Theological Studies,* 1956, **17**:332.

Ramsey, P. 1970: Ch. 4.

Sadler, A. et al. The Uniform Anatomical Gift Act. *JAMA,* 1968, **232**:2501.

Simmons, R., Klein, S. D., Simmons, R. L. *Gift of Life.* New York: Wiley, 1977.

Wolstenholme, G. E. W., O'Connor, M. (eds.). *Ethics in Medical*

* Complete citations for abbreviated references appear at the end of the book under "General References."

Progress: With Special Reference to Transplantation. Boston: Little, Brown, 1966.

4.3 *Confidentiality*

Beauchamp, Childress, 1979: Ch. 7.

Bok, S. *Lying: Moral Choice in Public and Private Life*. New York: Pantheon, 1978, Ch. 11.

Case Conference: The Limits of Confidentiality: Huntington's Chorea. *J Med Ethics,* 1976, **2**:28.

Cass, L. J., Curran, W. J. Rights of Privacy in Medical Practice. *Lancet,* 1965. (In Gorovitz, 1976: 82.)

Chayet, N. L. Confidentiality and Privileged Communication. *N Engl J Med,* 1966, **275**:1009. (In Gorovitz, 1976: 85.)

Davidson, H. A. Professional Secrecy. In E. Fuller Torrey (ed). *Ethical Issues in Medicine*. Boston: Little, Brown, 1968. (In Gorovitz, 1976: 87.)

Grossman, M. Confidentiality in Medical Practice. *Ann Rev Med,* 1977, **28**:43.

Marsh, F. H. The Deeper Meaning of Confidentiality Within the Physician–Patient Relationship. *Ethics Sci Med,* 1979, **6**:131.

Perkins, H. S., Jonsen, A. R. Conflicting Duties to Patients: The Case of the Sexually Active Hepatitis B Carrier. *Ann Intern Med,* 1981, **94**:523.

Smith, H. L. Professional Secrecy: A Vincible Right. *Linacre Q,* 1974, **41**:217.

Thompson, I. E. The Nature of Confidentiality. *J Med Ethics,* 1979, **5**:57.

Walters, L. Ethical Aspects of Medical Confidentiality. *Journal of Clinical Computing,* 1974, **4**:9 (in Beauchamp, Walters, 1978: 169).

Westin, A. New Era in Medical Records: Should Patients Have Access? *Hastings Center Report,* 1977, **7**(8):23.

Winslade, W. J. Psychotherapeutic Discretion and Judicial Decision: A case of Enigmatic Justice. In S. Spicker, H. T. Engelhardt, J. Healey (eds.). *The Law-Medicine Relation: A Philosophical Exploration*. Boston and Dordrecht: D. Reidel, 1981.

4.4 *Costs of Care*

Campbell, A. V. *Medicine, Health and Justice: The Problem of Priorities*. Edinburgh: Churchill-Livingston, 1978.

Campbell, J. D., Campbell, A. R. The Social And Economic Costs of End-Stage Renal Disease: A Patient's Perspective. *N Engl J Med,* 1978, **299**:386.

Carels, E., Neuhauser, D., Stason, W. *The Physicians and Cost Control*. Cambridge, Mass.: Oelgeschlager, Gonn & Haln, 1980.

Enthoven, A. C. Cutting Costs Without Cutting Quality of Care. *N Engl J Med,* 1978, **298:**1229.

Fried, C. Equality and Rights in Medical Care. *Hastings Center Report,* 1976, **6**(1):34.

Fried, C. Rights and Health Care: Beyond Equity and Efficiency. *N Engl J Med,* 1975, **293:**241.

Fuchs, V. *Who Shall Live?* New York: Basic Books, 1974.

Hiatt, H. H. Protecting the Medical Commons: Who Is Responsible? *N Engl J Med,* 1975, **293:**235.

McNerney, W. J. Control of Health Care Costs in the 1980's. *N Engl J Med,* 1980, **303:**1088.

Mechanic, D. Approaches to Controlling the Costs of Medical Care: Long and Short Range Alternatives. *N Engl J Med,* 1978, **298:**249.

Mechanic, D. Rationing Health Care. *Hastings Center Report,* 1976, **6**(1):34.

Pellegrino, E. D. Medical Morality and Medical Economics. *Hastings Center Report,* 1978, **8**(4):8.

Schwartz, W. B., Joskow, P. W. Medical Efficacy Versus Economic Efficiency: A Conflict of Values. *N Engl J Med,* 1978, **299:**1462.

Schroeder, S. A., Showstack, J. A., Roberts, E. H. Frequency and Clinical Description of High Cost Patients in 17 Acute Care Hospitals. *N Engl J Med,* 1979, **300:**1306.

Telfer, E. Justice, Welfare and Health Care. *J Med Ethics,* 1976, **2:**107.

Veatch, R. M., Branson, R. (eds.). *Ethics and Health Policy.* Cambridge, Mass.: Ballinger, 1976.

4.5 *Allocation of Scarce Resources*

Basson, M. D. Choosing Among Candidates for Scarce Medical Resources. *J Med Phil,* 1979, **4:**313.

Childress, J. Who Shall Live When Not All Can Live. *Soundings,* 1970, **43:**399–455. (In Reiser, Dyck, Curran, 1977: 620; in Shannon, 1976: 397.)

Gorovitz, S. Ethics and the Allocation of Medical Resources. *Medical Research Engineering,* 1966, **5:**5.

Outka, G. Social Justice and Equal Access to Health Care. *J Religious Ethics,* 1974, **2:**11. (In Shannon, 1976: 373; in Reiser, Dyck, Curran, 1977: 584.)

Rescher, N. The Allocation of Exotic Medical Lifesaving Therapy. *Ethics,* 1969, **79:**173. (In Gorovitz, 1976: 522.)

Siegler, M. A Physician's Perspective on a Right to Health Care. *JAMA,* 1980, **244:**1591.

Winslow, G. *Triage and Justice: The Ethics of Rationing Lifesaving Medical Resources.* Berkeley: University of California Press, 1982.

Weale, A. Statistical Lives and the Principle of Maximum Benefit. *J Med Ethics,* 1979, **5:**185.

4.6 *Research Values*

Annas, G. J., Glantz, L. H., Katz, B. F. *Informed Consent to Human Experimentation*. Cambridge, Mass.: Ballinger, 1977.

Feinstein, A. R. Medical Ethics and the Architecture of Clinical Research. *Clin Pharmacol Ther,* 1974, **15:**316.

Fried, C. *Medical Experimentation, Personal Integrity and Social Policy*. New York: American-Elsevier, 1974.

Hauerwas, S. Ethical Issues in the Use of Human Subjects. *Linacre Q,* 1978, **45:**249.

Hill, A. B. Medical Ethics and Controlled Trials. *BMJ,* 1963, **1:**1043. (In Reiser, Dyke, Curran, 1977: 278.)

IRB: A Review of Human Subjects Research. Hastings-on-Hudson, New York: Institute of Ethics, Society and the Life Sciences, published ten times yearly.

Jonas, H. Philosophical Reflections on Experimenting with Human Subjects. In Freund, P. (ed.). *Experimentation with Human Subjects*. New York: Braziller, 1969. (In Reiser, Dyke, Curran, 1977: 305–15.)

Jonsen, A. R. Ethical Aspects of Clinical Trials. *Triangle,* 1980, **19:**89.

Katz, J. (ed.) *Experimentation with Human Beings*. New York: Russell Sage, 1972.

Levine, R. J. *Ethics and Regulation of Clinical Research*. Baltimore: Urban & Schwarzenberg, 1981.

Levine, R. J., Lebacqz, K. Ethical Considerations in Clinical Trials. *Clin Pharmacol Ther,* 1979, **25:**728.

Lebacqz, K. Ethics and Clinical Trials. *J Cont Clin Trials,* 1980, **1:**29.

Lebacqz, K., Levine, R. J. Respect for Persons and Informed Consent to Participate in Research. *Clin Res,* 1977, **25:**101.

Protection of Human Subjects of Biomedical and Behavioral Research. Code of Federal Regulations Title 5. Public Welfare Part 46. *Federal Register,* **46**(16) January 26, 1981.

Schwartz, T. B. The Tolbutamide Controversy: A Personal Perspective. *Ann Intern Med,* 1971, **75:**303.

Shaw, L. W., Chalmers, T. C. Ethics in Cooperative Clinical Trials. *Ann NY Acad Sci,* 1970, 169:487.

Spiro, H. M. Constraint and Consent: On Being a Patient and a Subject. *N Engl J Med,* 1975, **293:**1134.

Stolland, J. F. Ethics of Clinical Investigators. *Am J Med,* 1979, **66:**554.

Walters, L. Some Ethical Issues in Research Involving Human Subjects. *Ethics Sci Med,* 1979, **6:**167.

4.8 *Social Considerations*

Badgley, R. F., Wolfe, S. *The Doctors' Strike: Medical Care and Conflict*. New York: Atherton Press, 1967.

Bowden, P. Medical Practice: Defendants and Prisoners. *J Med Ethics,* 1976, **2**:163.

Curran, W. The Ethics of Medical Participation in Capital Punishment. *N Engl J Med,* 1980, **302**:226.

Daniels, N. On the Picket Line: Are Doctors' Strikes Ethical? *Hastings Center Report,* 1978, **8**(1):24.

Derbyshire, R. C. Medical Ethics and Discipline. *JAMA,* 1974, **228**:59.

Dworkin, G. Strikes and the National Health Service. *J Med Ethics,* 1977, **3**:76.

Ethical Issues in Occupational Medicine. *Bull NY Acad Med,* Sept. 1975, **54**:No 8.

Sagan, L. A., Jonsen, A. R. Medical Ethics and Torture. *N Engl J Med,* 1976, **294**:1427.

Sissons, P. L. The Place of Medicine in the American Prison: Ethical Issues in the Treatment of Offenders. *J Med Ethics,* 1976, **2**:173.

CONCLUSION

This book has proposed the thesis that ethical decisions made by physicians should have, as their most decisive considerations, the medical indications for treatment and the preferences of the patient. The various sections of Chapters 1 and 2 have been attempts to show how these considerations can be applied to particular problems encountered in clinical practice. The thesis goes on to propose that considerations regarding quality of life and external factors become relevant only in quite particular circumstances. Chapters 3 and 4 have attempted to describe some of those circumstances. We hope this thesis and its applications will aid the practitioner in seeing complex problems more clearly and in evaluating how to act reasonably and responsibly in difficult situations.

GENERAL REFERENCES

Resources

Reich, W. (ed.). *Encyclopedia of Bioethics.* 4 vols. New York: Free Press, 1978.

Duncan, A. S. *Dictionary of Medical Ethics*. New York: Crossroad Publishing Co., 1981.

Sollito, S., Veatch, R. M. *Bibliography of Society, Ethics and the Life Sciences*. Hastings-on-Hudson, N.Y.: Institute of Society, Ethics and Life Sciences, issued annually.

Walters, L. (ed.). *Bibliography of Bioethics.* New York: Free Press,1981; issued annually.

BioethicsLine. National Library of Medicine Data Base. Medlars Management NCH. 8600 Rockville Pike, Bethesda, MD 20209.

Journals

The principal journals devoted exclusively or in large part to medical ethics are:

Bioethics Quarterly. Northwest Institute of Ethics and the Life Sciences. Human Sciences Press, 72 5th Ave., New York, N.Y. 10011.

Journal of Medical Ethics. Society for the Study of Medical Ethics. Tavistock House East. Tavistock Sq., London, WCIH 9JR.

Linacre Quarterly. A Journal of the Philosophy and Ethics of Medical Practice. The National Federation of Catholic Physicians Guilds. 850 Elm Grove Road, Elm Grove, Wis. 53122

Man and Medicine. Columbia University College of Physicians and Surgeons. 630 W. 168th St., New York, N.Y. 10032. (After Volume 6 [1981] retitled *Values and Ethics in Health Care*.)

Journal of Medicine and Philosophy. Society for Health and Human Values. University of Chicago Press. 5801 Ellis Ave., Chicago, IL. 60637.

Ethics in Science and Medicine. Pergamon Press. Maywell House, Fairview Park, Elmsford, N.Y. 10523.

Hastings Center Report. Institute of Society, Ethics and the Life Sciences. 360 Broadway, Hastings-on-Husdon, N.Y. 10706.

Anthologies and Collected Essays

Abernethy, V. (ed.). *Frontiers in Medical Ethics: Applications in a Medical Setting*. Cambridge, Mass.: Ballinger, 1980.

Bayles, M. D., High, D. M. (eds.). *Medical Treatment of the Dying: Moral Issues*. Cambridge, Mass.: Henkman, 1978.

Beauchamp, T. L., Walters, L. (eds.). *Contemporary Issues in Bioethics*. Encino, Calif.: Dickenson Publishing Co., 1978.

Gorovitz, S. et al. *Moral Problems in Medicine*. Englewood Cliffs, N.J.: Prentice-Hall, 1976.

Horan, D. J., Mall, D. *Death, Dying and Euthanasia*. Washington D.C.: University Publications of America, 1977.

Humber, J. M., Almeder, R. F. (eds.). *Biomedical Ethics and the Law*. New York: Plenum Press, 1976.

Hunt, R., Arras, J. (eds.). *Ethical Issues in Modern Medicine*. Palo Alto, Calif.: Mayfield, 1979.

Ladd, J. (ed.). *Ethical Issues Relating to Life and Death*. New York: Oxford University Press, 1979.

Reiser, S. J., Dyke, A. J., Curran, W. J. (eds.). *Ethics in Medicine: Historical Perspectives and Contemporary Concerns*. Cambridge, Mass.: MIT Press, 1977.

Robison, W. L., Pritchard, M. S. (eds.). *Medical Responsibility*. Clifton, N.J.: Humana Press, 1979.

Shannon, T. A. (ed.). *Bioethics*. New York: Paulist Press, 1976.

Williams, R. H. (ed.). *To Live and to Die: When, Why, and How*. New York: Springer, 1974.

Textbooks

Beauchamp, T. L., Childress, J. F. *Principles of Biomedical Ethics*. New York: Oxford University Press, 1979.

Bliss, B. P., Johnson, A. G. *Aims and Motives in Clinical Medicine.* London: Beckman, 1975.

Brody, H. *Ethical Decisions in Medicine,* 2nd ed. Boston: Little, Brown, 1981.

Campbell, A. *Moral Dilemmas in Medicine.* Baltimore: Williams & Wilkins, 1972.

Fletcher, Jos. Humanhood: *Essays in Biomedical Ethics.* Buffalo: Prometheus Books, 1979.

Fletcher, Jos. *Morals and Medicine.* Boston: Little, Brown, 1960.

Munson, R. *Intervention and Reflection: Basic Issues in Medical Ethics.* Belmont, Calif.: Wadsworth Publishing Co., 1979.

Ramsay, P. *Patient as Person.* New Haven: Yale University Press, 1970.

Smith, H. L. *Ethics and the New Medicine.* Nashville: Abingdon, 1970.

Vaux, K. *Biomedical Ethics: Morality for the New Medicine.* New York: Harper & Row, 1974.

Veatch, R. M. *Case Studies in Medical Ethics.* Cambridge, Mass.: Harvard University Press, 1977.

Warner, R. *Morality in Medicine.* Sherman Oaks, Calif.: Alfred Publishing, 1980.

Books and Resources in the Roman Catholic Tradition

Ashley, B. M., O'Rourke, K. D. *Health Care Ethics: A Theological Analysis.* St. Louis: Catholic Hospital Assn., 1978.

Healy, E. *Medical Ethics.* Chicago: Loyola University Press, 1956.

Kelly, G. *Medico-Moral Problems.* St. Louis: Catholic Hospital Association, 1953.

McFadden, C. J. *Medical Ethics.* Philadelphia: Davis, 1967.

O'Donnell, T. J. *Morals in Medicine.* Washington: Newman Press, 1957.

United States Catholic Conference. *Ethical and Religious Directives for Catholic Health Facilities.* Washington: USCC, 1971.

Books and Resources in the Jewish Tradition

Bleich, B. *Judiasm and Healing.* New York: KTAV Publishing, 1980.

Jakobovits, I. *Jewish Medical Ethics.* New York: Yeshiva University Press, 1972.

Rosner, F. *Modern Medicine and Jewish Law.* New York: Yeshiva University Press, 1972.

Rosner, F., Bleich, B. *Jewish Bioethics.* New York: Sanhedrin Press, 1979.

Tendler, M. *Medical Ethics: A Compendium of Jewish Moral, Ethical and Religious Principles in Medical Practice.* New York: Committee on Religious Affairs of the Federation of Jewish Philanthropies, 1975.